Just
Diagnosed
Breast Cancer

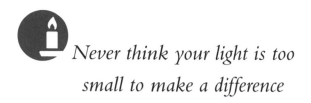 *Never think your light is too small to make a difference*

Arlene has hit this issue head-on and approached what can be a catastrophic event in a woman's life and turned her personal diagnosis into a testament of victory! So often women faced with breast cancer feel defeated and hopeless. After all, it's *our* breasts, an important part of who we are, and our feminine badge of honor is at stake! *Just Diagnosed* is the playbook of experience, fear, strength, and tenacity, a guide for all women who have faced breast cancer; may face breast cancer; or who need the confirmation that *I can, I will* take charge of my life, my breast, and survive! Arlene, I applaud you!
— **Hallia Baker,** *President, The Labor of Love Association Inc.*

This book fills an important void in consumer health literature. It takes the science of the breast cancer diagnosis and treatment out of the medical journals and streamlines it, making it accessible and understandable to everyday patients and their loved ones. As you read, you'll get the sense that Arlene isn't just dispensing information. Her approach is deeply human. She's your friend, your advocate, and, because she's walked this road before you, your Sherpa.
— **Steve Dunlop,** *communications trainer, former anchor and correspondent, Fox News and CBS News*

As a medical educator, Arlene has been a passionate and relentless force in bringing the most up-to-date information to the health-care community. She now brings that same relentless passion to educate and empower all of us through the breast cancer journey. Her words compel all to trust that inner voice and advocate for health and wellness. Her optimism makes survivorship possible.

— *Jean M. Cacciabaudo,* MD, FACC; FASNC;
   medical officer, Peconic Bay Medical Center,
   Northwell Health; assistant professor of Cardiology at
   Donald and Barbara Zucker School of Medicine at Hofstra/Northwell

---

Both informational and inspirational, this book is the goddess guide to the universe of breast cancer complexity. Few people have the grit and deeply inquisitive and tireless nature of Arlene Karole. With determination and courage to dig deeper, she's done the work and relieves the burden of "not knowing what to do." This well-organized stepwise guide helps readers prioritize not just their breast cancer-related consults and appointments, but to commit to greater awareness of what changes we can make to enjoy better health than what was "normal" before.

— **Ricki Pollycove,** MD, *San Francisco Integrative Gynecology*

In her own inimitable voice, Arlene Karole issues a deeply personal invitation into a breast cancer sisterhood that none of us choose but all of us cherish. Through wit and wisdom, anecdote and alchemy, she weaves practical advice, inspirational guidance, and deep caring intended to ease the burden of a breast cancer diagnosis. Arlene accompanies women on their journey as reluctant travelers on a feared and unknown path, helping them find the gift of deeper meaning along the way.

— **Laura Adams,** *special advisor, National Academy of Medicine;*
   breast cancer survivor

Just Diagnosed is at once a much-needed resource for those diagnosed with breast cancer and a deeply moving authentic exploration of one woman's universal healing journey. I look forward to offering this guide as a resource for my patients and to anyone in need of a comprehensive guide for navigating the breast cancer diagnosis. Arlene's uplifting attitude and positive self-agency permeates the book and, most important, helps anyone diagnosed with breast cancer feel they can handle the experience.

— **Lisa Langer,** *PhD, clinical psychologist; associate professor of Psychiatry at Donald and Barbara Zucker School of Medicine Hofstra/Northwell; Author,* Deeper into Mindfulness: Next Steps to Sustain Your Meditation Practice and Find Inner Peace; *certified Mindfulness-Based Stress Reduction (MBSR) teacher*

This book shares greatly helpful information for anyone facing a breast cancer diagnosis. Arlene's experience provides a clear benefit to those looking for help during one of the most difficult challenges in life. This book shares Arlene's experiences from the moment she heard those dreaded words—"You have cancer"—to today, where she has come full circle and is now a volunteer for the Breast Cancer Helpline at SHARE, the same helpline that aided her through her own ordeal.

— **Christine Benjamin,** *LMSW; SHARE, senior director, Patient Services and Education*

This inspirational book about Arlene's own experience and journey provides the reader with detailed research and guidance in how to advocate for yourself through this sensitive topic. Its writing is aided by her New York wit and personality. Having known Arlene for almost eight years, she has always demonstrated a passion and drive to serve others through her work and personal life. Listening to her body was pivotal in empowering herself during her experience, which led her on this path of determination to know more about this devastating diagnosis—and how it almost was missed.

— *Tracy Lin,* PT Cert.; MDT; RYT-200, *advanced clinician physical therapist, Mount Sinai Medical Center*

Just Diagnosed is a must read for patients who have received a breast cancer diagnosis, as well as one for their families and caregivers. A brilliant woman with extensive knowledge of a large health system's intricacies and complexity, Arlene's inspiring story is one of empowerment, advocacy, and hope.

— *Ann C. Lichti,* CHCP; FACEHP;
  Vice President of Outcomes, Accreditation, and Compliance, PER, Physician's Education Resource, LLC

Just as the Vinnie Myers Team provides a unique service to survivors in need of closure, Arlene Karole provides a unique service to her "breast friends" with this enlightening collection. Her facts, figures, and fighting mentality will rally those just starting their journey and those looking for answers.

— *Vinnie Myers,* tattoo artist,
  Vinnie Myers Team and *Little Vinnies Tattoos*

Arlene has been a friend and colleague for twenty years; this book reminds me why our friendship has lasted. She is insightful and speaks in a voice we can understand and believe. While supporting her views with helpful information, she tells a compelling and relatable story that will undoubtedly aid many women in her shoes. While I would expect nothing less from this talented author, I continue to be amazed by her drive, skills, and knowledge. Arlene speaks from the heart; it is our privilege to listen.

— **Rick Amari,** *founder, Columbus Consulting Inc.*

Having worked with Arlene for many years, I have found her passion, enthusiasm, and innovative teaching create a dynamic learning environment that allows her students to thrive both inside and outside the classroom. With this approach mirrored in *Just Diagnosed*, she guides her readers with warmth and candor, offering many teachable moments. With commitment and authenticity, she provides her readers a how-to guide for taking ownership of and navigating their diagnosis.

— **Glenn Gerstner,** *PhD; MBA; Dean, The Lesley H. and William L. Collins College of Professional Studies, St. John's University*

"Know…
You *are* loved.
You *are not* alone.
Everything *is* possible.
There is *always* hope.
You got this!"

— *Arlene M. Karole, CHCP*

Just
Diagnosed
Breast Cancer

What to Expect
What to Know
What to do Next

**A candid collection of information
you can use on your journey to healing**

ARLENE M. KAROLE, CHCP

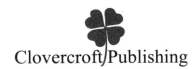

Clovercroft Publishing

Just Diagnosed: Breast Cancer
What to Expect What to Know What to do Next

©2021 by Arlene M. Karole, CHCP

Published by Clovercroft Publishing, Franklin, Tennessee
www.clovercroftpublishing.com

Page xxiv: Quote: Ralph Waldo Emerson,
https://www.goodreads.com/quotes/357811-to-know-even-one-life
Page 86: Quote: Oliver Wendell Holmes, Jr.,
https://www.goodreads.com/quotes/9241174-a-mind-that-is
-stretched-by-new-experience-can-never
Page 142: Quote: Ralph Waldo Emerson, https://www.goodreads.com/
quotes/15579-what-lies-behind-us-and-what-lies-before-us-are

Content Edits by Robert Irvin

Technical Edits by Conor Greene, PA-C

Editorial Services and Interior Design by Adept Content Solutions
www.adeptcontentsolutions.com

Front Cover Design and Layout Consulting by Francesca Lum
Lum & Associates • www.lumassociates.com

Back and Spine Cover Design by Suzanne Lawing

Photography by Beowolf Photography www.beowulfsheehan.com

Sam Salerno at Reel Media www.reelmedia.tv/about

ISBN: 978-1-950892-82-2

Printed in the United States of America

Contents

Contents

ICONS USED IN THIS BOOK

MINI MENTION

These are side notes that expand on topics and sometimes insights from influencers (messengers) who came into my life at just the right time to make a positive and essential impact on the choices I made.

DEFINITIONS

These are medical terms that may be related to your diagnosis, names of associations that may help you in your journey to healing, or detailed information on references I make in the book.

My Promise to You, My Reader

While our life experiences and life journeys, much like our diagnoses, may be unique, inside at our very core, at our very essence, we are all the same. We are human beings. We are all striving to be and do our very best in our time here on this planet.

My promise to you is to the best of my ability through my personal experience with breast cancer, show you too how you can become empowered and take control of and own your diagnosis and not have it own you.

While there is much information out there on breast cancer, seek out that which is based on science (evidence-based). In this book I will share a collection of information and resources that I came across during my journey that may help you as you embark on yours. This is a starting point.

My promise to you is to the best of my ability to guide you through my personal experience and share the knowledge I have gained to give you a head start on making the most informed decisions you may very well begin having to make, right now, in this moment in time, from your diagnosis forward.

To My Ancestors

Who immigrated and voyaged from Poland and Ireland, for without their struggles and determination to start anew in America—*we would not be.*

My mom, journaler, avid lover of English and history, who listened without judgment and always gave of herself most lovingly and unconditionally.

My dad, World War II veteran and pilot, architect, artist, and motivator.

Sophie and Alexander, Honora, and Thomas
For having vision and persevering, we are grateful.

It is from *you all* who were before us we have inherited our strength, courage, and determination to keep moving forward.

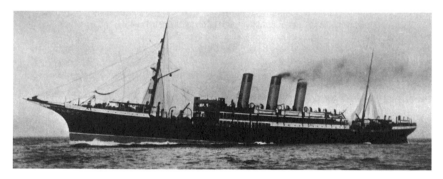

My grandmother, Sophie Drewnowska, arrived at Ellis Island, New York, on September 14, 1906. When eighteen years old, she left Poland and sailed aboard the SS *Smolensk*, shown above. She immigrated to America seeking refuge from persecution and economic hardship. *Photo courtesy of Kevin Blair.*

For My Mom, Rita,

Thank you for giving me wings.

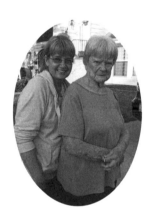

"If there's a book that you want to read, but it hasn't been written yet, then you must write it."

—*Toni Morrison*[1]

Preface

Quite honestly, this book came about by pure accident. So, in part, I've called it my accidental book. But the fact is, I personally don't believe in pure accidents or chance or luck. Now that's not saying that while I may be destined to live to age 101, if I choose to walk in front of a bus, well, clearly, I may not make it to 101. The point is, while we do have control of our actions, I believe we are also in the hands of . . . whatever you want to call it, him, or her—*the divine, the universe, or God.* There are many wonderful opportunities in life, as well as burdens, that come our way, and they do so in all shapes, sizes, varieties, trials, and challenges. It's *our choice* to take what we are given and make something of it.

And so it was early on in my diagnosis, in my research, in March 2015, that I came across the *Cancer Research UK Science Blog,*[2] and it haunted me. It read:

> Only a small proportion, about one in 20 (5 percent) of the 50,000 women diagnosed with breast cancer every year carries an inherited gene fault like BRCA1. Most breast cancers arise from genetic damage that accumulates over a person's lifetime; that's why age is the biggest risk factor.

I wondered: *Why? When? How?* Would my genes be damaged over the course of my lifetime? We have longevity in our family tree, no breast cancer in the family, no BRCA gene—aka the *breast cancer gene*—and yet I had been diagnosed with breast cancer. It was those few sentences from the *Cancer Research UK Science Blog*, in part, at least, that provided the fuel that kept me digging and digging for answers to the many questions that ultimately led from one chapter to the next.

In March 2020, while I was attending Mass, there were a couple of lines in a hymn I heard that struck me and made me think of my breast cancer, my breast friends, and those *just diagnosed* with breast cancer. The lines were these:

> This journey is our destiny. Let no one walk alone. The journey makes us one.[3]

Breast cancer, I have come to find all these years later, is a lifelong journey, and while my diagnosis was devastating, it is now having gone through it that I am able to share with you my experience in the hope of making yours a little easier.

And the truth is—while looking back at my first notes typed in June 2015, if I had the chance to go back to March of that year when I was just diagnosed and receive a different diagnosis, one that would change my having to get a mastectomy of my right breast, *I would not change a thing.* This book is my way of paying it forward. This opportunity to do something good with what was to be my destiny, my misfortune, unluckiness, or whatever you want to call it, is truly my honor and privilege. This allows me to share my experiences to give hope and empower you on your journey. *For that I am full of gratitude.*

THE STATE OF HEALTHCARE IN THE UNITED STATES TODAY

When reading and watching the news and listening to discussion in general on healthcare, it always blows my mind that the United States spends more on healthcare[4] than any other high-income country, yet we have the lowest life expectancy and the highest suicide rate among wealthy nations.

The Centers for Disease Control (CDC) reports the top ten leading causes of death in the United States,[5] with heart disease ranked first and cancer trailing right behind at second with over 1.2 million Americans diagnosed with either disease, and the list of other illnesses goes on from there. With that I ask, how can it be that our country, which strives to make our health and healthcare a top priority, is in such poor health?

We are bombarded with billions of dollars from companies marketing, promoting, and messaging us on how to live better while we spend our hard-earned dollars trying to live healthy lifestyles—joining gyms and weight loss programs, exercising more, eating better foods, eating less food—and yet we are still not living our absolute best.

While overall in the past four decades heart disease and cancer have been declining,[6] they are still our nation's top two killers. Again, I wonder with all this money and focus spent on getting healthy, where are all these diseases coming from? *How are we as consumers contributing to the problem or, at the very least, not doing a better job at keeping ourselves healthy—body, mind, and spirit?*

Yet, despite all these diseases, at least until very recently, we have been living longer. For example, the female life expectancy in 1930[7] was 61.6 years of age; in 1965, for those just on the cusp of being baby boomers (born 1946–1965), life expectancy had risen to 73.8.[8] By 2017 the average life expectancy for a female had risen to 81.2[9] (with men's life expectancy trailing some years behind). However, while we are living longer, are we *living better?* Are we living what I call our absolute best?

While my initial research started out with wanting to understand more about my breast cancer diagnosis, as one step led to another unexpected step and yet to another (as many did along this journey), I came across numerous reports, studies, and opinion pieces not directly associated with breast cancer (and hard to overlook) that addressed other prevalent diseases in our society, our wellbeing as it relates to our emotional and mental health, and national crises in our country that affect public health as well as our social and economic welfare.

One report in particular stood out. It was by The Commonwealth Fund and titled "Mirror, Mirror on the Wall, 2014 Update: How the U.S. Health Care System Compares Internationally." The report's executive summary notes:

> The United States health care system is the most expensive in the world, but this report and prior editions consistently show the U.S. underperforms relative to other countries on most dimensions of performance. Among the 11 nations studied in this report—Australia, Canada, France, Germany, the Netherlands, New Zealand, Norway, Sweden, Switzerland, the United Kingdom, and the United States—the U.S. ranks last, as it did in the 2010, 2007, 2006, and 2004 editions of Mirror, Mirror. Most troubling, the U.S. fails to achieve better health outcomes than the other countries, and as shown in the earlier editions, the U.S. is last or near last on dimensions of access, efficiency, and equity.[10]

In its 2017 update, the report highlights in its opening paragraph how the United States is still falling far short. An excerpt:

> The United States spends far more on health care than other high-income countries, with spending levels that rose continuously over the past three decades. Yet the U.S. population has poorer health than other countries. Life expectancy, after improving for several decades, worsened in recent years for some populations,

aggravated by the opioid crisis. In addition, as the baby boom population ages, more people in the U.S.—and all over the world—are living with age-related disabilities and chronic disease, placing pressure on health care systems to respond.[11]

And in its 2020 update, particularly alarming, it noted that U.S. suicide rate is the highest among wealthy nations.[12]

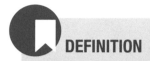

DEFINITION

THE COMMONWEALTH FOUNDATION HISTORY[13]

Among the first private foundations started by a woman philanthropist, Anna M. Harkness, it was established in 1918 with the broad charge of enhancing the common good.

The mission of The Commonwealth Fund is to promote a high-performing healthcare system that achieves better access, improved quality, and greater efficiency, particularly for society's most vulnerable, including those with low income, the uninsured, minority Americans, young children, and elderly adults.

The Fund carries out this mandate by supporting independent research on healthcare issues and making grants to improve healthcare practice and policy.

An international program in health policy is designed to stimulate innovative policies and practices in the United States and other industrialized countries.

I came across an article in *Fortune*[14] by Grace Donnelly: "Here's Why Life Expectancy in the U.S. Dropped Again This Year." This article notes that for the second year in a row, life expectancy for Americans dropped, to 78.7 years, according to the CDC's National Center for Health Statistics—putting the United States behind other developed nations and 1.5 years lower than the Organization for Economic Cooperation and Development (OECD), where the average life expectancy is 80.3 years.

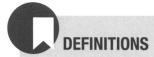

DEFINITIONS

THE ORGANIZATION FOR ECONOMIC COOPERATION AND DEVELOPMENT (OECD)[15]

The OECD is an intergovernmental economic organization, with thirty-six member countries, founded in 1961 to stimulate economic progress and world trade.

BRITISH MEDICAL JOURNAL (BMJ)[16]

A weekly peer-reviewed medical journal and one of the world's oldest general medical journals of research, clinical practice, and healthcare policy since 1840 for general practitioners, hospital doctors, and educators.

The article goes on to share a new study published by the *British Medical Journal (BMJ)* titled "Failing Health of the United States,"[17] which looks in to the broader cause behind the decline in life expectancy and found ... despair. Dr. Steven Woolf, and associate professor of emergency medicine at the Virginia Commonwealth University and coauthor of the report, said, "We are seeing an alarming increase in deaths from substance abuse and despair."

According to the National Institute of Health (NIH): National Institute on Drug Abuse, 128 people die every day from an opioid overdose.[18] Reading the *BMJ* study and watching the video included in the article—"Ground Zero for the

Opioid Crisis,"[19] which highlights a county in West Virginia where more of the population is dying from prescription pills than motor vehicle accidents—is heartbreaking on so many levels. Dr. Woolf added that the amount of the decrease in life expectancy[20] is actually less alarming than the fact that addiction and a decline in the emotional wellbeing of Americans have been significant enough to drag down the country's average length of life.

Furthermore, a joint panel of the National Research Council and Institute of Medicine, determined to study why America's new life expectancy,[21] 78.7 years, falls so far below the OECD average of 80.3, found a wide variety of contributing factors, from obesity and diabetes to homicides and HIV/AIDS.

So, while my initial research started out in search of answers to learn more about my breast cancer diagnosis, I started to have more questions than answers and started seeing some overall alarming trends and themes in our lack for our own care of self. I started to think about the word *disease* and what it really means by definition. And I started to think about the undertones of how disease can possibly manifest itself in our bodies not just in the physical sense but emotionally and spiritually as well.

As I have experienced firsthand—and you may too—hearing the words "you have cancer" is no better motivator to then start looking inward and reevaluating your life. Those quiet moments alone with ourselves and being introspective are most difficult but enlightening. I found myself asking questions like, "What could I have maybe done differently? Was I a contributor to my own illness?" And I found myself now serendipitously on a journey evaluating many other areas of my life and the choices I had made thus far.

The United States is one of the richest, freest, and most blessed countries in the world; how is our healthcare the worst among eleven industrialized countries?[22]

- What responsibility do companies have?

- What responsibility do our employers have?

- What responsibility do our pharmaceutical companies have?

- What responsibility does our federal government or states have?

And importantly, what is *our* responsibility to ensure we are better informed and to take better care of ourselves?

It is all these questions—and so many more—and digging and digging for answers that led to this "accidental book."

"One's philosophy is not best expressed in words; it is expressed in the choices one makes . . . and the choices we make are ultimately our responsibility."

—*Eleanor Roosevelt*[23]

"To know even one life has breathed easier because you have lived. This is to have succeeded."

—*Ralph Waldo Emerson*

Part One
The Journey Begins

"Everything can be taken
from a man but one thing:
the last of the human freedoms—
to choose one's attitude
in any given set of circumstances,
to choose one's own way."

—*Viktor Frankl*[1]

Chapter One
Just Diagnosed

S o here I was, at forty-nine . . .

Who would have thought that instead of planning for my fiftieth birthday on August 14—designing invitations and figuring out guest lists with my good friend Paula, graphics designer extraordinaire—I'd be planning for a mastectomy of my right breast? Really!

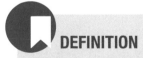

DEFINITION

MASTECTOMY[2]

A mastectomy involves the surgical removal of all of the breast tissue. In many instances, much of the breast skin and even the nipple can be spared. A mastectomy is typically recommended for women who have multiple areas of cancer and/or large tumors relative to the size of the breast. There are several different types of mastectomy[3]:

- **Nipple-sparing mastectomy:** only the breast tissue is removed;

- **Skin-sparing mastectomy:** the breast tissue is removed with the nipple and areola;

- **Total (simple) mastectomy:** the breast tissue and skin are removed;

- **Modified radical mastectomy:** the whole breast is removed, along with the lymph nodes under the arm.

I feel great! I feel strong! I look beaming healthy! Working out at the gym four times a week (okay, really three times), so … surgery? How long will that take? ! I'm busy!

At 5:45 p.m. on a Friday evening in April on the Long Island Railroad, I was on my way back to Manhattan from my office in Great Neck, Long Island, when my cell phone rang. I picked it up and heard, "Ms. Karole?" I answered, and the next thing I heard was "You need to schedule a CT chest scan, a right axilla lymph node biopsy, and an MRI breast biopsy." Caught completely off guard, all I could say was, "What?!" After a few other comments, she said, to sum it up, "Your MRI lit up," and they needed more tests. Almost to Penn Station, entering the tunnel to Manhattan and about to lose cell reception, I said thank you and ended the call. Needless to say, I didn't have time to ask: Additional tests for what? I feel great! I feel strong! I'm full of energy!

I had all weekend to research, and bottom line, when I typed in "MRI lighting up," it was like a punch in the gut! I was alarmed and shocked to see all of the articles and links that popped up that were tied to breast cancer. Really? *Breast cancer?* But my two mammograms and one ultrasound were "normal." *I'm sure this will be fine … right?*

Action Items

Action Items

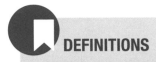

DEFINITIONS

MAGNETIC RESONANCE IMAGING (MRI)[4]

Magnetic resonance imaging (MRI) is a test that uses a magnetic field and pulses of radio wave energy to make pictures of organs and structures inside the body. In many cases, an MRI gives different information about structures in the body than can be seen with an X-ray, ultrasound, or computed tomography (CT) scan. An MRI may also show problems that cannot be seen with other imaging methods.

For an MRI test, the area of the body being studied is placed inside a special machine that contains a strong magnet. Pictures from an MRI scan are digital images that can be saved and stored on a computer for more study. The images can be reviewed remotely, such as in a clinic or an operating room.

In some cases, contrast material may be used during the MRI scan to show certain structures more clearly. You may be able to have an MRI with an open machine that doesn't enclose your entire body. But open MRI machines aren't available everywhere. The pictures from an open MRI usually are not as good as those from a standard MRI machine. The resolution is lower, giving the radiologist less information to make an accurate assessment.

MRI is an excellent tool to detect breast cancer. Cancerous growths enhance or "light up" on breast MRIs. Unfortunately, many noncancerous abnormalities may enhance as well. To diagnose a cancerous lesion that is only seen on MRI and not felt or seen on a mammogram

Action Items

Action Items

CHAPTER ONE

or ultrasound, and sometimes in order to distinguish between a cancerous and benign (noncancerous) lesion, a biopsy may be needed.

False Positives[5]

Breast MRIs can pick up things that other imaging techniques can't, such as those mammograms and ultrasounds do not. MRIs are probably the most sensitive of the imaging techniques. MRIs have a lot of false positives, which means your MRI can light up, signifying the presence of cancer, but it can be something as simple as inflammation. MRIs can show a lot of things that are *not* cancer, sometimes leading to unnecessary further testing. In the simplest of terms, a false positive indicates that a given condition is present in the body when it is not.

CT CHEST SCAN[6]

A CT scan is an X-ray technique that gives doctors information about the body's internal organs in two-dimensional slices, or cross-sections. Your doctor might order CT scans to examine other parts of the body where breast cancer can spread, such as the lymph nodes, lungs, liver, brain, and/or spine.

Currently, CT scans are not routinely used to evaluate the breast. If you have a large breast cancer, your doctor may order a CT scan to assess whether the cancer has moved into the chest wall. This helps determine whether the cancer can be removed with mastectomy.

Action Items

Action Items

AXILLA LYMPH NODE BIOPSY[7]

A lymph node biopsy is the removal of lymph node tissue for examination under a microscope. The lymph nodes are small glands that make the white blood cells that fight infection. Lymph nodes may trap the germs that are causing an infection. Cancer often spreads to lymph nodes.

IMAGE GUIDED BREAST BIOPSY[8]

This procedure takes a sample of suspicious tissue from inside your breast, with the help of radiologic imaging. A biopsy can be performed using ultrasound, mammography, or MRI.

The procedure is pretty much the same either way. Your radiologist numbs the area with local anesthetic, and with the help of the imaging machines, a probe is inserted into the breast to remove some of the abnormal tissue. A small titanium marker is placed inside the breast to mark the area that is sampled. Finally, a pathologist will examine the specimen under a microscope to determine a diagnosis.

So here is my situation: we have no cancer or breast cancer in the family. Well, okay, my beloved and favorite aunt, Hedy, who died of natural causes at ninety-three, did have some form of breast cancer. Already in her late eighties, she was at a checkup at her cardiologist when they discovered it but chose to leave it alone due to her age.

How I found out about Aunt Hedy's breast cancer was after being asked the same exact question *over and over* again

Action Items

Action Items

on multitudes of forms I filled out before each new doctor's appointment. "Do you have a history of breast cancer in the family?" I didn't think so and had never heard about it, but I wanted to be sure, so I asked my mom and then found out.

Frankly, on both sides of our family, for the most part, we are in great health and live well into our late eighties and nineties. Clearly, we have good genes, *right?*

MINI MENTION

So I have to stop here and comment as I found myself asking many obvious questions: Why me? Why now? And . . . how? I too stumbled into and upon issues I never dreamed I would think about on my journey with breast cancer.

It was on this journey, for the first time in my life of forty-nine years that I understood what the phrase "ignorance is bliss" meant. And I discovered that while we may be born with a great gene pool, the foods we eat, the air we breathe (I worked in the Ground Zero zone on and after 9/11), our attitude, and even the way in which we carry ourselves throughout our day and practice living don't necessarily guarantee that our genes will stay that way.

I—at least, until I received my diagnosis of breast cancer—never stopped to think how my everyday choices could possibly impact my health. You may now, having been just diagnosed, want to take account and reflect on your personal choices over the years.

ACTION ITEMS

ACTION ITEMS

So seeing those two words—*breast cancer*—when I initially researched the words "MRI lighting up," well, I thought that would be the most powerful punch to my gut, the most shocking, the most frozen-moment-in-time feeling I'd have.

Boy, was I wrong.

Early on in my diagnosis, when I was headed for a second opinion at a medical center in New York—that was the hardest punch yet. While my primary care doctor and the other doctors I had seen were always on the east side, it was for this particular visit that I was told to go to an office in midtown. I was like, *Hm, I wonder what building that is.* I've never seen any of my doctors at this particular location. On the day of my appointment, I knew I was getting close as I saw their very defining logo on the building facade in the distance. As I got closer, I could read the wording, and I was immediately sick to my stomach and horrified: Cancer Center! *Why am I at a cancer center? I don't have cancer! Or . . . do I?* You just simply can't believe it is happening to *you!*

AND SO THE JOURNEY HAD BEGUN! AND HERE ARE SOME BASIC THINGS I QUICKLY FOUND OUT

Trust Your Gut

While I was told by most physicians that "breast cancer does not resonate with pain," it was that simple little pinprick on my right breast and slight ache under my right armpit—infrequent and nonalarming as it was—that made me go, *Hm, get it checked out early on.* Ladies, please listen to and know your body and take action!

Action Items

Action Items

Be Persistent!

It was after having two mammograms and one ultrasound that I was told in writing and in person "everything's normal." It was my pure persistence and saying to my doctor as I was literally walking out of her office, "I'm telling you something's just not right, but if you say it's okay, then okay." With my hand literally on the door handle, she spoke up.

"Wait!" she said. "If you don't need an authorization for an MRI, let's do an MRI." I did not need an authorization—*thankfully.*

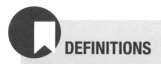

DEFINITIONS

MAMMOGRAPHY[9]

Mammography is an X-ray imaging method used to examine the breast for the early detection of cancer and other breast diseases. It is used as both a diagnostic and screening tool. There are two main types of mammography: film-screen mammography and digital mammography.

ULTRASOUND[10]

Ultrasound is an imaging test that sends high-frequency sound waves through your breast and converts them into images on a viewing screen. The ultrasound technician places a sound-emitting probe on the breast to conduct the test. There is no radiation involved.

Ultrasound is not used on its own as a screening test for breast cancer. Rather, it is used to complement other screening tests. If an abnormality is seen on

ACTION ITEMS

ACTION ITEMS

mammography or felt by physical exam, ultrasound is the best way to find out if the abnormality is solid (such as a benign fibroadenoma or cancer) or fluid-filled (such as a benign cyst). It cannot determine whether a solid lump is cancerous, nor can it detect calcifications.

So the same thing, ladies: don't ignore your gut or a symptom, and if you feel something, say something! Don't let it go. And make sure if you feel you need to get a second, a third, or as many medical opinions as you like, then do it! Take control of your diagnosis; don't let it take control of you!

 MINI MENTION

So I have to stop here and share something else I feel is important.

I thought: *What if I do need an authorization for the MRI test?* With three tests—both mammograms and an ultrasound—showing no disease and having no breast cancer in the family, my doctor said the insurance company likely would not authorize the need for an MRI. I thought, *Would I have paid out of pocket for this test that's much more expensive than a mammogram?* Honestly, I likely would have held off.

Then I think about what we found on that MRI when it lit up, which ultimately showed extensive, eight to nine centimeters of ductal carcinoma in situ (DCIS), or Stage 0, not yet technically considered cancer (so they said)—could it have spread? Could it have

ACTION ITEMS

ACTION ITEMS

turned into invasive cancer, which is considered *now really* cancer? And the answer, according to one doctor, was yes, it could have. So, thankfully, I did not need an authorization for that MRI. But think of those who may!

Through my research I found actress Christina Applegate was diagnosed with breast cancer in 2008 at the age of thirty-six. Like my diagnosis, hers went missed by the traditional mammogram and ultrasound. It was only after she got an MRI that she received the devastating news that she had full-blown breast cancer. Initially she underwent a lumpectomy, but after learning that she had the BRCA genetic mutation, she chose to have a double mastectomy. Ms. Applegate has since started an outstanding foundation, Right Action for Women, which offers MRI assistance.

Thus, the MRI is extremely important in helping to identify a disease that other tests—certainly in my and Ms. Applegate's case—missed. However, due to the high cost of the MRI and for other reasons, unless there's a prior confirmation of disease, insurance companies may not pay for it.

Which leads me to ask, how are our health "insurers" insuring our health? Who's really got the power to make *our* healthcare decisions about what tests we should or shouldn't get? Our doctors? The government? Corporations looking out for their own profit margin? Or how about—maybe—*we* know our own bodies and take action? Just sayin'!

ACTION ITEMS

ACTION ITEMS

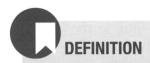

DEFINITION

DUCTAL CARCINOMA IN SITU (DCIS)[11]

DCIS is the most common type of noninvasive breast cancer. *Ductal* means that the cancer starts inside the milk ducts, *carcinoma* refers to any cancer that begins in the skin or other tissues (including breast tissue) that cover or line the internal organs, and *in situ* means "in its original place." DCIS is called noninvasive because it hasn't spread beyond the milk duct into any normal surrounding breast tissue. DCIS isn't immediately life threatening, but having DCIS can increase the risk of developing an invasive breast cancer later on in that same breast. When you have had DCIS, you're at higher risk for the cancer coming back or for developing a new breast cancer on that breast than a person who has never had breast cancer before. Most recurrences happen within five to ten years after initial diagnosis.

Regardless of the controversy of whether DCIS is considered cancer or not, nearly 20 percent of all breast cancer cases are DCIS, with more than 60,000 cases diagnosed each year. In situ cancers are more prevalent among women in their forties and fifties and plateau after age 60.

Do Your Research

It was then, during the MRI lighting up, that we found something. We found eight to nine centimeters of DCIS. As one doctor said, "It's a miracle this was found." Another said, "This is the best diagnosis you can wish for." However, not

ACTION ITEMS

ACTION ITEMS

13

CHAPTER ONE

one surgeon would rule out a mastectomy due to the extensive number of unhealthy cells found in my right breast. But I found myself replaying their words in my head and trying to find comfort. I thought to myself, *Well, if this is the "best diagnosis," which entails cutting off my right breast, what is the worst diagnosis?*

Again, here is my action item: research, research, research! You will be faced with myriad new terminologies coming at you and having to make choices, including types of surgery and reconstruction—or not—that will be available to you. But let me be clear: the doctors will not tell you what to do, at least not one of mine did. They can only lay out the possible treatments for your case and give their best opinion. Look for resources that are reputable and fact- and evidence-based.

Be Knowledgeable

Unfortunately, as with the initial two mammograms and one ultrasound, my two MRI breast biopsies missed the invasive cancer cells lurking in my breast tissue. Remember, I had about eight to nine centimeters of disease, and each biopsy only takes a tiny piece of tissue, a few millimeters, usually. They found preinvasive disease but not the invasive part! *Only after I chose* to have a mastectomy did they find 3.5 millimeters of, yes, invasive cancer. Thus, they now staged my breast cancer as Stage 1A.

So, here, a caution: whether talking to physicians, breast friends, or doing research, there's a tremendous amount of information available to us, and to an extent, some is conflicting. On this journey I was told by one doctor at a top hospital in New York, "In medicine, nothing's 100 percent." Be knowledgeable. Know your options. There will still be questions, but exhaust

Action Items

Action Items

all efforts, and then you will know that the action you take is ultimately best for you!

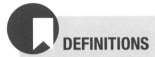

DEFINITIONS

INVASIVE BREAST CANCER[12]

The most common invasive breast cancer is **invasive ductal carcinoma**[13]—abnormal cells that come from the ducts of the breast, the tissue acting as channels for milk to leave the body. These account for about 80 percent of breast cancers. The other most common invasive cancer is **invasive lobular carcinoma.**[14] This one arises from the lobules of the breast, where breastmilk is formed. There are other rare subtypes like **mucinous carcinoma, medullary carcinoma,** and **tubular carcinoma**[15] to name a few, but they are generally quite rare and don't differ much in terms of treatment from the more common types.

In any invasive cancer, the abnormal cells have broken through the original structure and begun to move into new areas, usually those next to the disease.

BREAST CANCER STAGING, SIMPLIFIED[16]

Stage 0 is DCIS, as noted above.

Stage I describes invasive breast cancers that are invasive but still relatively small—smaller than two centimeters and with no or little disease in lymph nodes.

Stage II disease is a bit larger, somewhere between two to five centimeters of disease, and usually accompanied with disease in one to three lymph nodes in the axilla.

ACTION ITEMS

ACTION ITEMS

Stage III can be any size and often includes disease that has spread to or involved with the skin of the breast, as well as the axillary lymph nodes.

Stage IV disease is a tumor of any size that has spread to distant organs.

WHAT'S IT LIKE FOR OTHERS?

As I continued on this journey, what weighed on my mind, was thinking about others who:

Maybe didn't pay attention to their symptoms. I wondered: how many other people felt the same pinprick or another physical sensation and had the same "normal" breast imaging, and went a year (or more!) without treatment? Did their cancer spread?

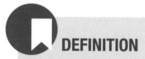

DEFINITION

METASTASIS[17]

The spread of cancer cells from the place where they first form to another part of the body. In metastasis, cancer cells break away from the original (primary) tumor, travel through the blood or lymph system, and form a new tumor in other organs or tissues of the body. The new metastatic tumor is the same type of cancer as the primary tumor. For example, if breast cancer spreads to the lung, the cancer cells in the lung are breast cancer cells, not lung cancer cells.

Didn't have an understanding about the healthcare system that, as patients, we are thrust into. What about those who

Action Items

Action Items

didn't maybe have that little extra access that I had to doctors since I work as an educator in a health system? How did their journey go? Even with a little extra knowledge and access, *it isn't easy.*

Perhaps don't have access to proper health insurance for their doctor visits, treatments, or tests, let alone the second or more opinions they may want to have. Or, I thought—as I may have foregone that first MRI due to cost—did they make that choice? What was their outcome?

Are older or maybe not in the best of health—those who just don't have the energy or stamina or knowledge to fight to be their own "healthcare advocate." What happens to them? It can be absolutely exhausting to manage the scheduling of endless doctor appointments, tests, and surgeries, especially if still working a full-time job and juggling life's other priorities—and to look as though you are keeping it all together!

Yes, I found myself thinking about those others, and in the beginning, those like me, who didn't know *how* or *whom* to ask for help, embarrassed and not wanting to admit to myself or others I was sick. Yes, I found myself thinking about those who were *just diagnosed* and who, like me, had *no idea* what lay ahead!

HOW DID THIS BOOK COME ABOUT?

It was my awesome mom, Rita, and amazing friend Anita who were among the first I told about my breast cancer diagnosis. I couldn't believe it. It was only by "chance," when I was headed to my first appointment, that, separately, both Mom and BFF

Action Items

Action Items

Anita told me to "make sure you take notes!" I thought, *There shouldn't be many notes to take! This will be quick; I don't have breast cancer. Do I?* (And yes: deny, you will.) I brought a pen and some sticky notes.

The doctor appointments started to mount, and those sticky notes and few pieces of scrap paper ran out. I would then ask the girls behind the desk if they could give me some white copy paper from their office printer. (We do what we have to do! I'm not shy.) Then I started to bring my own copy paper!

On the top of each piece of paper I would write the name of the doctor I was meeting with, the date, and the time of our appointment. I would write up the same questions for each appointment, and this helped me accurately compare the doctors' answers from each appointment. Looking back, this was my way of beginning to gain control of my diagnosis! And this should be yours too.

I'm a very visual person, and as the notes continued to mount, I found the need to highlight things, so then I began toting colored markers along with me. Then the single sheets of paper became many, and I started to staple them all together. I ran through many pens! I then brought a notebook until, finally, it was too much information scattered all over the place. I just wanted it all in one centralized location.

So I started to type up my notes from all those sticky notes, scraps of paper, copier paper, and the notebook—all into one Word document on my computer. And it was during one moment, sitting there quietly at my computer, overwhelmed from the amount of notes I had accumulated, that the reality began to hit home: I had breast cancer, right? And it was in that moment that I realized I had written sixty-three thousand words!

Action Items

Action Items

WHY I CHOSE TO WRITE THIS BOOK

These sixty-three thousand words became my guide. They became invaluable as I navigated my way on this journey. These notes helped me keep track of the tremendous amount of information that was coming at me and helped me make my *best* choices and decisions for what type of surgery and procedures and reconstruction would be best for me. It was also at this moment, as I stared at my sixty-three thousand words, that I called my long-time business coach and friend Alexandra and said, "Alexandra I just wrote sixty-three thousand words. What do I do with this?" And she said I must share my experience to help others and that my sense of advocacy was powerful and to break it down into chapters and keep it simple. And that's what I did.

I am writing this book for *you*! For those of you just diagnosed with breast cancer. And also for your family, friends, and colleagues who will need to be aware and understand what your journey ahead may hold—and how to help get you through it in the best way possible. Through sharing my personal journey with you, I hope to make your journey a little easier.

I am writing to let you know I have been overcome by warmth, kindness, and unconditional love and inducted into a sisterhood I never knew existed. *And you will be too.* Writing about my journey and sharing it with you is my way of paying it forward. Know you do and will have support and you are *not alone.*

When searching for advice and guidance, I have found women don't hesitate to talk to me about anything. They all— and I mean *all*—simply listen and openly share their journey, a journey I frankly didn't realize I was on, but somehow *they did.* As I continued to seek my own guidance, I talked with women

Action Items

Action Items

from different life experiences and ages, and I came to realize breast cancer has no borders, and it does not discriminate by age or gender or race, by social or financial status, by celebrity, or by how high you get on the career ladder.

I am writing to let you know you can get through this! You *will get through this*, but you have to take charge of your diagnosis, and you must stay strong.

I am writing to be a guide for you; really, going into my journey, I didn't have one. I will share resources and information that were a great help to me in hope they will help you. And I'll address issues and questions you may be too embarrassed to ask, would never think to ask, or would never have thought you'd need to ask!

And if you have not yet realized it, this is now your number-one priority, and you must play an active role in getting yourself healthy. I want you to know that while I had excellent doctors and phenomenal healthcare—and you will have the best for you—*you* are ultimately the person who must make your decisions that you will have to live with the rest of your life! Doctors will *not* tell you what to do. You will have to make the final decisions.

I believe in all of us: we have a connection to our higher power, that inner voice, and we can access it. We simply have to be still and listen. And there is no better time be still and listen than after hearing those three words "you have cancer." Yes, listen to your inner voice, your gut, your conscience, your body. As it was exactly that *listening*, that *feeling*, that . . . *knowingness* . . . that occasional "pinprick" in my right breast above my nipple that led me to be persistent and allowed me to catch my disease early.

Action Items

Action Items

Throughout this journey I was graced by many supportive family, friends, colleagues, and furry friends, and you will be too. Just weeks before my scheduled surgery, and still conflicted about the procedure, I had a "serendipitous" opportunity to speak with a prominent doctor on the West Coast. I happened upon her because she was a faculty member of an educational program I was working on in New York. After reaching out to her for advice and guidance as I shared with her my diagnosis, she warmly said, "You've joined a sisterhood." Ironically, it was a sisterhood, I was coming to find, that everyone knew I had joined before I did! I was in denial, as you likely will be too. *You never think it will happen to you.*

I am writing to acknowledge those "breast friends," a term I came up with by chance when trying to categorize my new friends. My breast friends are women and men who helped me from across the globe—from Paris to Toronto to the west and east coasts of the United States—who, not knowing anything about me other than I was referred through a friend of a friend to talk with them about their experience and journey, from that first call, or that first email, immediately showed me the greatest unconditional love and, with full and open arms, welcomed me into the sisterhood.

Just when I was resigned to removing my breast and yet still holding out, still *hoping* this would all just go away, now just weeks before my scheduled mastectomy, my mom called me. She said, "I just saw a doctor on television talking about breast cancer, and she's the chief breast surgeon at a well-known hospital." Now, I'd been to that hospital, and that doctor's name was not on the door. I thought, *How many more doctors can I see? I'm done.* But then that nagging feeling of hope came over me:

ACTION ITEMS

ACTION ITEMS

What if she's the one who will tell me this isn't cancer and I don't have to remove my breast?

She did not, thankfully. And the very next day I was in her office along with my wonderful friend Anita! The doctor spent almost two hours with us. Now mid-May and two months since my diagnosis back in March, it seemed like an eternity had passed. It was here at this very last appointment, for the first time, that I *cried*. I realized this was it.

I was going to have a mastectomy in two weeks.

"Learn to get in touch with the silence within yourself and know that everything in this life has a purpose, there are no mistakes, no coincidences, all events are blessings given to us to learn from."

—*Elisabeth Kubler-Ross*[18]

ACTION ITEMS

ACTION ITEMS

NOTES

"You gain strength, courage, and confidence by every experience in which you stop to look fear in the face."

—*Eleanor Roosevelt*[1]

Chapter Two
The Journey Begins: Owning Your Diagnosis

I schedule annual visits to my primary care doctor, gynecologist, dermatologist, dentist, and so on (and you should too!). Like clockwork, I go for my annual mammogram. Every year leading up to and including 2015—February 2015, to be precise, from which these journaling notes came—I received the standard letter I was accustomed to receiving in the mail. It read, as usual, "We are pleased to inform you that the results of your breast exam performed on [date] are normal. It is recommended that you have your next routine screening breast exam in one year." All good.

Oddly, I had been feeling a pinprick-like feeling in my right breast above my nipple. It was infrequent at first, happening maybe every few weeks, so I did not pay it much attention. And then it happened a few more times. In addition to that pinprick feeling (literally like someone taking a pin and pricking my skin with it), I would also have an occasional ache under my right armpit. But again, I wrote that off, thinking that maybe I just stretched too much while doing a downward dog in yoga class.

Until it happened a few more times. Again, this is so vital: pay attention and listen to your body!

I was headed back to the gynecologist. She asked if I drank a lot of coffee. Guilty! She said, "Try rubbing primrose oil on your breast and cut back on the coffee." Hm. Really? Okay. So I bought the primrose oil and rubbed it on daily. I must confess I was not giving up my coffee, though I did cut back and switched a few cups to decaf. But that pinprick and that ache continued. At the gynecologist office a couple of weeks later, she did one last physical exam. Finding nothing, she suggested I see a breast surgeon.

Taking her advice, I immediately made an appointment with a breast surgeon. Accessing my electronic health records (EHR), the new surgeon I was seeing, now mid–March, reminded me I had just had a mammogram in February and that it was "normal." I said, "Yes, however," and I went on to explain the strange pinprick feeling on my right breast and the ache under my right armpit. So she ordered a second mammogram. This test too showed "normal." My mammograms back in March and August of 2014 were "normal" too! Done in two different hospitals. Hm.

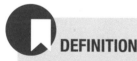

DEFINITION

ELECTRONIC MEDICAL RECORD (EMR)[2] AND ELECTRONIC HEALTH RECORD (EHR)[3]

An EMR contains the standard medical and clinical data gathered in one provider's office. An EMR is a digital version of a paper chart that contains all a patient's medical history from one practice. An EMR

Action Items

Action Items

is mostly used by providers for diagnosis and treatment. The information stored in EMRs is not easily shared with providers outside of a practice. A patient's record might even have to be printed out and delivered by mail to specialists and other members of the care team.

EHRs go beyond the data collected in the provider's office and include a more comprehensive patient history. EHRs are designed to contain and share information from all providers involved in a patient's care. EHR data can be created, managed, and consulted by authorized providers and staff from across more than one healthcare organization.

Unlike EMRs, EHRs also allow a patient's health record to move with them—to other healthcare providers, specialists, hospitals, nursing homes, and even across states.

The point of mentioning EMRs and EHRs is if you go for a second opinion, you will likely be asked to share with your new doctor your prior test results. So before you go through the process of heading to the medical records department—a long, arduous task—check to see if your doctors' practices have these digitized software systems.

As I pressed on with her and talked about the strange pinprick, she said, "Breast cancer doesn't present with pain." Most other doctors I met with said the same. I say again, *listen to your own body and be persistent.* If you feel something is not right, it very well may not be. I was persistent. Be persistent! Wouldn't you rather know if something maybe is not right

ACTION ITEMS

ACTION ITEMS

and address it early on than *wait and see*? Yes. I knew you would agree!

She recommended I get an ultrasound. They found, yet again, nothing; everything was "normal." I lay on that table in the ultrasound room as the radiologist did the test, rolling the ball around on my breast with that clear sticky cold gel (hopefully they warm it up for you!). And she had said, confidently, "There is nothing here."

It was at that very point, after reviewing the test results of my two mammograms and one ultrasound with my breast surgeon and once again reviewing the ultrasound report with the radiologist—and being told "there are no unusual or suspicious findings"—that I said to my breast surgeon, "Okay, I'm done. If you say it's nothing, okay!"

Even though I *knew* something did not feel right, I felt a bit embarrassed and frankly hard pressed to continue to persist when an accomplished surgeon with extensive credentials—and three linchpin tests—all said there was nothing wrong with me. You may feel the same! *But do not let it go!*

As I was walking out of her office with my hand on the handle and the door half-opened, my doctor said, "Okay, wait. If your insurance does not need an authorization for an MRI, we will get you in for an MRI." My insurance carrier thankfully did not need authorization.

It was that first call I received at 5:45 p.m. on the Long Island Railroad, as my doctor's office called to tell me my MRI lit up and I needed to schedule three additional tests, when I found strength and courage. It was *instinctive*. I flew into survival mode (is there any other mode to be in?) *And you will and must too.* I knew I had to get on and tackle this. Being a person of faith, I prayed as well—a lot. And of

ACTION ITEMS

ACTION ITEMS

course I felt great, I looked healthy, and I was sure this was nothing.

I would go on to need a CT chest scan, a right axilla lymph node biopsy, and an MRI-guided breast biopsy. I thought, *Why in the world would I need a chest scan? And what does a lymph node have to do with this? What is a lymph node? And how are these three tests connected?*

I had all weekend to research, and research away I did. I learned quite a bit about breast cancer that weekend. I learned that, like any cancer, as breast cancer invades tissue, it may begin to spread to other parts of the body. The lymph nodes of the axilla tend to be the first place breast cancer spreads to, followed by other sites like the lungs, liver, bones, or even the brain if left untreated. With that pinprick feeling resonating on my right breast, I now understood the need for a biopsy and CT scan. It was extremely scary to realize breast cancer can spread to so many places. So I now found great motivation to address the issue and do so quickly!

 MINI MENTION

As an admitted type A personality, well, in part, those qualities served me well in my breast cancer journey. I quickly organized myself and mobilized a strategy to find out what I had, and, being assertive, I scheduled doctors' appointments and tests in record time. But let me be clear it was also done reluctantly and, truly, I did not want to face this diagnosis. *But what was the alternative?*

I prepared for surgery and visited my mom in Staten Island a week before—to prep the house and bring

Action Items

Action Items

over my belongings and my furry friends. I planned to stay there for a couple weeks post-surgery as my mom would help me begin my recovery.

After my immediate diagnosis I was overwhelmed and didn't get to connect with everyone in the manner in which I would have liked. But that day in Staten Island I passed by Cheryl's house, a childhood friend, and I popped in to see her. She brewed some coffee and we sat down to catch up. I shared my news.

Cheryl listened quietly. While normally she would have said something, looked shocked, or had some reaction, she was, I thought, eerily quiet. *Hm.* But I kept talking.

Finally, she shared that her sister-in-law, who I knew well from having attended family gatherings over the years, three months earlier struggled with a backache. Cathy, a busy and successful executive, popped some pain meds and figured her back pain would go away.

Until it continued to worsen over the next several months. Finally, my friend shared that her brother, Cathy's husband, finally said, "You're going to the doctor." She went. It was at that initial appointment, at the young age of fifty-two, that she was diagnosed with Stage 4 breast cancer that had metastasized into her spine, causing the severe back pain. Cathy had extensive surgeries over the course of the next two years. She died in September 2017.

I cannot emphasize this enough, ladies: if you feel something is not right, go to the doctor! *Do not wait and see.*

ACTION ITEMS

ACTION ITEMS

So now I was armed with some knowledge of what I might have. Bright and early Monday morning, I was on the phone scheduling those tests. Of course, this was much ado about nothing, right? I would get it behind me quickly and get back to planning my fiftieth birthday party.

Unfortunately, that was not to be the case. It is overwhelming as you're scheduling these tests and appointments all the while processing the fact you may have breast cancer, and you're trying to go about your day like everything is fine!

MINI MENTION

Let me stop to mention a few more important things.

CONFIRM YOU HAVE INSURANCE APPROVALS

There are many insurance carriers out there, and each has different rules and requirements when it comes to testing. As I shared, thankfully in my case my insurance carrier did not need a prior authorization for my MRI. I confirmed this with my doctor's office a few days prior to my MRI. But if the insurance company did require an authorization, and by chance I went ahead with the test not having that authorization, they likely would not have paid for it.

I learned along my journey that while the doctor's office is likely (supposed to) to check and call for authorizations and mostly do (since they want to be paid), there were a few near misses leading to extra anxiety and stress, and this you do not need.

Action Items

Action Items

Here again, while doing the best they can, you must make *sure*, prior to your tests, lab work, X-rays, and more, that you have all approvals from your health insurance company. Having the approval in writing is optimal. An email or verbal confirmation works too. However you get it, make sure you record the name of the person you spoke with, the date, the time, and the authorization number. This will be of great value; if there is an issue you have your notes!

Hopefully your doctor's office will help you coordinate this and call you a day or two prior to confirm insurance details, but do not count on that: be proactive! Otherwise, you can end up paying a very expensive bill—or arguing about it for months.

CONFIRM WITH THE DOCTOR'S OFFICE THAT ALL ANCILLARY SERVICES ARE COVERED IN YOUR INSURANCE PLAN

As I've found along the way, even though I confirmed my doctors were 100 percent covered under my insurance plan, they would then send me for testing in laboratories for blood work or to a radiologist for X-rays that were *not covered* under my insurance.

How do you prevent this from happening? Make sure, after arriving for your visits, to tell the receptionist to note your record (they can do that), and to tell the doctors. And as with confirming your insurance approvals, also make sure you note the date, time, and names of whom you spoke with sharing that these ancillary services *must* be covered and billed within your insurance

Action Items

Action Items

plan or you're not responsible for paying the bill! That should resonate.

But even with that, I still had to battle some bills with billing departments—but I prevailed. Why? I had dates and names of those I documented this with.

I know you're exhausted; I was too, and overwhelmed. But be prepared!

ASK QUESTIONS! LOTS OF QUESTIONS! AND SPECIFICALLY: WHY AM I TAKING THIS TEST?

Make sure *prior* to your tests or lab work you ask, "Do I need to do anything to prep for this test?" And understand why you are taking it and what exactly it is for. Number one: you should know. I recall on a few tests I showed up thinking, *What is this for?* I was exhausted, but that's no excuse. Be informed: this is your health. Take the time! Number two: on a couple of occasions, I showed up for tests where, on one, I was not supposed to eat after midnight the night before, and for another test I was not supposed to have my period within seven days of having the test. Thus, hearing about this the morning of—the person booking the tests *forgot to tell me*—we had to reschedule, wasting everyone's time and adding to my stress level.

Do your due diligence. Ask questions!

SECURE YOUR TEST RESULTS

I urge you to make sure to get copies of *all* your test reports, X-rays, lab work, pathology slides, CDs, and the paper reports that accompany them. You want these

Action Items

Action Items

for your records to keep track of exactly what you are taking and the results for the short-term as well as for the future. If you go for another opinion, that doctor will likely ask you for all prior tests and results for their review.

I came to find my breast doctor's office was a revolving door of patients! They are busy, and you will likely be waiting for your test results to first get to your breast surgeon and then find yourself waiting for your breast surgeon's office to contact you. In almost all cases I'd get the reports before the doctors did. It's not that hard, but it is time consuming; be both diligent and proactive in your own care. *I know you will!*

While the chest CT scan showed a small nodule, it was normal. A nodule can form, I was told, simply by having coughed excessively during a cold, thus forming scar tissue—a form of nodule—on your lungs. One down!

The right axilla lymph node biopsy also was normal, meaning there was no disease found in my right underarm lymph node. Thus, if disease was present, it had not spread. Two down!

The MRI-guided breast biopsy, well, that was a different story. The first biopsy showed extensive ductal carcinoma in situ (DCIS), and the second biopsy showed other areas that were "highly suspicious" for more DCIS. DCIS is considered Stage 0 breast cancer and is the most common type of noninvasive breast cancer. It is called noninvasive since it hasn't yet spread beyond the milk duct into any surrounding breast tissue. However,

ACTION ITEMS

ACTION ITEMS

DCIS can become invasive breast cancer. And here is the key point: *in my case it did.*

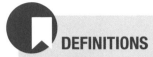

DEFINITIONS

NODULE[4]

A nodule is a growth of abnormal tissue. Benign pulmonary nodules can have a wide variety of causes. Many are the result of inflammation in the lung resulting from an infection or disease producing inflammation in the body. The nodule may represent an active process or be the result of scar tissue formation related to prior inflammation.

LYMPH NODE[5]

Any of the small bodies located along the vessels of the lymphatic system (in humans notably in the neck, armpits, and groin) that filter bacteria and foreign particles from lymph fluid. During infection, lymph nodes may become swollen with activated lymphocytes.

And so with both the first and second biopsy confirming the extent of disease in my right breast (done April 2015), I received a voicemail on my cell phone, which I still this have saved on my phone, from my breast surgeon. In summary, she shared, "One area was more DCIS and another area was highly suspicious for DCIS, and we've documented over eight centimeters, and I really think you need a mastectomy, as I suspected. And I think you need to meet with the plastic surgeon." *Gasp!* I'm like, *The plastic surgeon? For what?*

Action Items

Action Items

Thinking back, it was like each doctor's appointment, each test, each phone call, each *everything* was leading me slowly, painfully, step by step where I did not want to go: to the truth. *I have breast cancer. Really?!*

MINI MENTION

For those of you who may have just gasped yourself and may even be incensed at hearing my doctor confirm I may need a mastectomy by leaving me a voicemail on my cell phone, the truth is, texts and cell messages were the quickest and easiest way for me and my doctor to communicate. You too will need to convey to your doctors how you would best like to communicate.

It is far and few between, understandably, that you will get your doctors on the phone, given their busy patient and surgery schedules. Doctors, like us, are overworked and working within the limitations of our everchanging and somewhat strained healthcare system.

I wanted to know all my test results immediately; I didn't want to play phone tag. Frankly, often I'd have my test results and lab reports before my doctor even called me! I wanted to be on top of my diagnosis, and by the time she called, I had questions ready for her.

That said, I will admit that particular message was jarring to hear for the first time: you may need a mastectomy! Regardless, my doctor is amazing. Through this entire journey she kept seamless and open communication with me via texts at any time I texted and through phone and all office visits.

Action Items

Action Items

THE FIRST MEETING WITH THE PLASTIC SURGEON

When going to meet with the plastic surgeon for the first time I brought my gal pal Anita; she accompanied me on almost every doctor appointment. We were escorted into his office and seated at his large, beautiful mahogany desk and told, "He'll be right in."

It was while sitting there, quietly, waiting, looking around at his impressive and many degrees on the wall, family photos, and various books on the shelves, we both looked down and, *yes!*—there before us, lying forth on this beautiful mahogany desk, were three boobs!

Now I don't want to sound completely ignorant; we identified them as breast implants! But to see your potential new body part lying there in front of you on a desk, I have to tell you, I was like, *Really!* Anita, who's usually most direct and expressive, was absolutely speechless. And her lack of expression and comments made me think, *Wow, this is really serious.*

 MINI MENTION

Once more I need to stop and share.

Ladies, make sure you identify, and have with you at your doctors' appointments, one smart cookie! In addition to yourself, of course. Make sure to bring a friend, a family member, a coworker—*someone* who will help think with and for you. *You will be overwhelmed.* It will be important to have someone alongside you who will be looking out for you, someone to ask the questions you didn't think to ask, are too exhausted to think about, or too scared to hear the answers to!

Action Items

Action Items

Like me, you may find yourself in the midst of myriad emotions. From disbelief and denial (and rightfully so, by the way; we never expect "this" will happen to us) to feeling strong and hopeful (that I would change my own diagnosis) to complete sadness and powerlessness, it will be a roller coaster of emotions. At least it was for me, down to that very last doctor's appointment in May, just weeks before my surgery. Hang in there! You will get through this. How do I know? Because I was in your shoes, and I did.

It was at this initial consultation the surgeon sat with us for more than ninety minutes and talked about different options for breast reconstruction surgery. He discussed the benefits and drawbacks of both breast implant and deep inferior epigastric artery perforator (DIEP) procedures.

BREAST IMPLANTS

There was no way I was going to have some foreign material in my body. I just couldn't imagine what that might feel like. And is it healthy? But then again, I was there with a diagnosis of breast cancer! That plastic surgeon went on to say that breast implant surgery was less invasive, shorter in duration, and just as likely to provide a good cosmetic result. However, the implants need to be replaced every ten to fifteen years, your body may reject them, and due to scar tissue forming, they may harden. Hm.

Breast implants have a bad reputation among some women who aren't familiar with how far the technology has come. I

ACTION ITEMS

ACTION ITEMS

only ever thought of implants as something women got for cosmetic reasons, never realizing they were commonplace in reconstruction surgery. When my surgeon brought them up, I thought how in the eighties there were some health concerns with implants. Breast implants at the time had thinner shells and much more liquid silicone than is used today. I thought about an issue I had heard implants have with leaking or breaking. There is a higher rate of capsular contracture (scar tissue around the implant causing it to feel firm and look distorted) with the implants we use today.

However, due to innovation and technology and overall advances in healthcare, we have come a long way, and they are very safe and a welcome alternative for women who may not have another feasible option.

With that said, as you'll read on in the next chapter, "Breast Friends," I heard directly from women who have implants, and they shared that they look and feel natural, and they are happy with their decision versus choosing another procedure that was also an option for them. And for various reasons, not everyone will be a candidate for deep inferior epigastric artery perforator (DIEP) flap. I encourage you to do your own research on the benefits and risks of all options that will be made available to you and your unique diagnosis.

DEEP INFERIOR EPIGASTRIC ARTERY PERFORATOR (DIEP) FLAP

He then discussed the DIEP procedure. This initially appealed greatly to me as here you use your own body tissue to build a new breast! He went on to share they do not have to be replaced, there is no real chance of rejection as you are using

Action Items

Action Items

your own body tissue, they are natural, and as a bonus, you get a tummy tuck. However, the surgery is more complicated, requiring longer operative and hospitalization time, and there is a 1 to 2 percent chance of necrosis, or the death of localized tissue and failure of the graft.

With this exchange, the meeting in his office was ended. He then asked me to head to the exam room, get in a gown, and have the opening to the front. Anita asked, "Do you want me to come?" I was like: *I'm certainly not going in there alone!* It was here he opened the gown and was looking full frontal. Talk about *cringe.* I thought, *I really should have lost that five . . . ten . . . okay, fifteen pounds!* So he continued to "assess." He finally spoke and said, "Well, it looks like you are eligible for the DIEP procedure." So basically, for this surgery, they take fat from your belly and build your new breast out of your own fat and tissue. I had a fairly simple thought: *Kind of amazing, cool, and gross all at the same time!*

Who knew? Yes, *who knew* that having been unsuccessful the last six months in trying to get that pudge off my belly, those few pounds—okay, fifteen—that my belly fat would come in handy? I thought, *Wow. God has a plan for everything.* I was excited about the *bonus* tummy tuck until I understood what that procedure entailed: a hip-to-hip incision across your abdomen. *Hm.* I thought I'd rather hit the gym! Just sayin'. The surgeon proceeded to take photos from the front and side. Again, *cringe.* It's so awkward and embarrassing. But, rest assured, this too will pass. You will get over this quickly.

For a first appointment, this was a tremendous amount of information to process—and completely unnerving. The bottom line is there's no easy way to talk about breast reconstruction

Action Items

Action Items

that may take place after a mastectomy. I appreciated the surgeon's sensitivity, the time he took with us, and his directness. He was direct and needed to be. That actually helped me confront my diagnosis.

I think Anita, my friends, and family all had thought this would be just fine. But truly that appointment was the crossing-over-the-bridge moment as both Anita and I walked out of that appointment absolutely speechless. Needless to say, I started to have more questions than I had answers.

By the way, while first planning on the DIEP procedure, I changed my surgery plan just days before. I chose ultimately to get reconstructive surgery with a breast implant for my right breast, and to balance out my breast size, they also put an implant in my left breast to even everything out. Lastly, I chose to remove my nipple. Not knowing whether it had disease lurking in it but still wanting to keep as many of my body parts as possible, days before surgery I called a good friend of mine and shared my dilemma with her. She quickly shot back, "Arlene, why would you leave an old part on a new car?" And thus too removed my nipple. More on this all later.

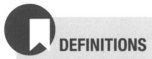

DEFINITIONS

DEEP INFERIOR EPIGASTRIC ARTERY PERFORATOR (DIEP) FLAP[6]

DIEP is the technique where skin and tissue (no muscle) are taken from the abdomen in order to recreate the breast. The surgeon grafts the harvested tissue to your breast by connecting the breast's native blood supply to

Action Items

Action Items

the blood vessels in the harvested tissue. Here fat, skin, and blood vessels are cut from the wall of the lower belly and moved up to your chest to rebuild your breast. In a properly performed DIEP, no muscle is cut or removed; if you're having DIEP flap, make sure this will be the case. Your surgeon carefully reattaches the blood vessels of the flap to blood vessels in your chest using microsurgery. Because no muscle is used, most women recover more quickly and have a lower risk of losing abdominal muscle strength.

SALINE BREAST IMPLANTS[7]

These are filled with sterile salt water. They're inserted empty and then filled once they're in place. Saline breast implants are available to women eighteen and older for breast augmentation and to women of any age for breast reconstruction.

SILICONE BREAST IMPLANTS[8]

These are prefilled with silicone gel, a thick, sticky fluid that closely mimics the feel of human fat. Most women feel that silicone breast implants look and feel like natural breast tissue. Silicone breast implants are available to women twenty-two and older for breast augmentation and to women of any age for breast reconstruction.

ACTION ITEMS

ACTION ITEMS

NIPPLE-SPARING[9] AND SKIN-SPARING MASTECTOMY[10]

For a nipple-sparing mastectomy, your surgical oncologist and plastic surgeon will be able to preserve your original nipple, areola, and overlying skin while still removing all the breast tissue and reconstructing a breast. In skin-sparing mastectomy, the nipple is removed but more of your original skin can be left behind than in a typical mastectomy. Not everyone is a candidate, however. The size or amount of disease present in the breast, as well as how close that disease is to your skin or nipple, will determine the best course.

TAKE CONTROL AND OWN YOUR DIAGNOSIS; DON'T LET IT OWN YOU!

Instinctively, I knew I had to be strong and moving forward addressing this diagnosis seriously. But at the same crazy time, I'm thinking, *I'm sure this is nothing, this is going to go away, and everything will be fine, right?* But it was not going to go away. I reluctantly looked fear in the face. I looked! We have to! Any of you just diagnosed can and will do the same. I know this because I was there; I was in your shoes.

So *how* did I take control, find strength, and look fear in the face, you may ask. The same way you will: *by owning and taking charge of your diagnosis.*

I've identified seven steps that helped me and hopefully will help you too! You can access them in **Resource A: 7 Steps to Own and Take Charge of Your Diagnosis.**

Action Items

Action Items

43

Here are a few thoughts to get you started!

Take notes from that initial appointment forward as you meet with your doctors. Take *scrupulous* notes highlighting dates, times, doctors, or others you met with and items discussed.

Patient education is key. Learn about breast cancer and its various stages, identify the type you have, and be clear on your individual diagnosis, treatment options, and so forth. There is a *lot* of information out there. Go to the best sources that are science- and evidence-based, well-known, and trustworthy. I've included many that I've found extremely helpful in the resource section of this book. Talk to family members. Is there a history of breast cancer in the family?

Research new terminologies your doctors may discuss with you, and ask them to explain these to you. The time for questions is while you are there in front of them in their office. There's no calling them afterward to chat. While my doctors are amazing, I also came to learn their offices arc like revolving doors of breast cancer patients they see all day long. A mastectomy, by definition to them, is commonplace. To me, I was like, *What?!* So be sure to ask a lot of questions. Do your research ahead of your appointments. Go prepared. I cannot stress this enough.

Whether you are doing your research at the local public library, on your home computer, at work on your lunch break, reading books, or speaking with others, be informed. Exhaust all possibilities *and yourself* in the process until you are completely satisfied with the answers so you can make the most informed and best decisions possible with no regrets!

Ask! Whether it be the meaning of the tests or procedures you're being told to have or why exactly you're having a particular

ACTION ITEMS

ACTION ITEMS

test or procedure, ask. Ask! Do these tests have risks? If there are associated risks, what are they? Do the benefits outweigh the risks?

How—or *do?*—these tests relate to one another? Know your doctors' credentials and specific areas of practice in relation to your specific diagnosis and surgery. Ask! How many procedures like the one you are scheduled to have do they do perform per week? Per month? You do not want anyone practicing their technique on you!

For example: While I was originally scheduled for the DIEP surgery, through my careful research I learned that a plastic surgeon doing this procedure should have training in microsurgery, critical for that particular surgical procedure. Mine did.

As we were taught in school, no question is silly—this definitely holds true now. And frankly, I asked anyway! It's *your* health, *your* money, and *your* time!

MINI MENTION

The absolute need and reason to ask questions couldn't have become clearer for me early on. At some point after my MRI-guided breast biopsy, I received an X-ray. As usual I had to begin to train myself early to get a copy of all my tests from the medical records department.

As I was looking at one X-ray, I noticed a silver-looking piece of something on the film, maybe the size of a tee-ny-tiny bird seed. I was told it was a "titanium marker" left in my body. I was like, *for what?* It was left as a marker as to where they pulled the cells from. This way if they pull another sampling, it will be from another area. This is an

ACTION ITEMS

ACTION ITEMS

example I share with you to add to the long list of things *no one tells you.* That's why you must do your own research.

I was so beyond annoyed by this. Why was I annoyed, you may ask. I thought that this was all going to be over soon and now I had a piece of metal left in my body they didn't even tell me they would leave there. *Can they get it out? Will it move? Can it go off on airport detectors?* (They did, it doesn't, and it can't—not that I knew, that though.) All these thoughts were crushing into my head! I wanted it removed. Anyway, it did get removed—along with all my breast tissue during my mastectomy! Again, ask questions!

Financial support. Perhaps you may need insurance coverage, help with copays, or support for transportation, housing, out-of-pocket, or other medical or ancillary expenses. If you have health insurance, make sure to call your insurance company and ask what doctors are covered under your plan. Whatever your needs, research, then reach out!

I've identified some resources for you that provide support in these areas. This is just a start. There are many amazing organizations out there to help you! You can access them in **Resource F: Organizations That Provide Helpful and Exceptional Support.**

You are going to own your diagnosis by being an informed consumer! That's how you are in control. Ultimately you are a customer and healthcare is a business, and *your* business is taking care of you! Gear up! This is a lifelong journey and know *you are not alone.*

ACTION ITEMS

ACTION ITEMS

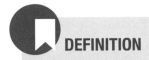

DEFINITION

X-RAY[11]

An electromagnetic wave of high energy and very short wavelength that is able to pass through many materials opaque to light.

A photographic or digital image of the internal composition of something, especially a part of the body, produced by X-rays being passed through it and being absorbed to different degrees by different materials.

So it was getting clearer to me that—after meeting with a primary care doctor, a gynecologist, breast surgeons, and plastic surgeons, then after numerous mammograms, ultrasounds, MRIs, a CT chest scan, and a right axillary lymph node biopsy followed up with MRI-guided breast biopsies (all, by the way, done in record timing of twelve weeks from diagnosis to my surgery on Wednesday, June 10—be persistent!)—this was to be the beginning of what would become a yearlong—or should I say lifelong—journey!

From your first doctor appointment, test, and diagnosis forward, here's the short list of likely medical professionals, departments, providers, and individuals you may need or want contact with and should begin to identify early on.

- Billing department

- Breast surgeon

- Clinical care coordinator/patient navigator (bridging the gap between patients and processes)

- Medical records

Action Items

Action Items

- Oncologist (you may want to discuss with your doctor the need to see an oncologist prior to surgery)
- Pathology department
- Spiritual support provider (priest, minister, rabbi, imam, etc.)

I've identified a comprehensive list for you. You can access both **Resource B: Medical Professionals and Spiritual Support Providers** *and* **Resource E: Beyond Your Doctors.**

MINI MENTION

I have to stop here and say whichever doctor's office and/ or department you are visiting with, become familiar with all frontline office staff at the desk. I made sure to get names, emails, and phone numbers. Sometimes I brought flowers and goodies. These ladies and men will become very familiar faces as they are the amazing team members manning the front office desk, who may book your appointments, get your medical authorizations, help you navigate the system, *and more.* Like us all they work hard, and a little thank you or appreciation goes a long way!

DEFINITION

CLINICAL CARE COORDINATOR OR PATIENT NAVIGATOR[12]

What is a care coordinator? Although they have many names—care coordinators, transplant coordinators, nurse coordinators, nurse navigators, patient navigators—they

Action Items

Action Items

all have the same purpose of bridging the gap between patients and processes.

While each person's experience and diagnosis are unique, I share this list with you to prepare you for what to expect on your journey, to identify early on the proper and countless departments and individuals you may need to coordinate with. Navigating through "the system" is daunting, and being prepared is imperative.

An acknowledged type A personality, while I have personally always struggled with the virtue of patience, it is on this journey with breast cancer that you will need to push forward while maintaining and demonstrating a great deal of patience. Patience for yourself, patience for the healthcare team you choose and staff you will be in contact with, and patience with many others. Plan to hunker down and stay fully engaged, steady, and moving forward. Truly and literally, from your first test and initial diagnosis to your surgery to post-recovery, this is a step-by-step process. We all—patients and healthcare workers—have to work within and navigate our somewhat strained healthcare system. Patience at this time truly will be a virtue.

MY LAST APPOINTMENT WITH MY BREAST SURGEON BEFORE SURGERY

So, down to the wire, literally twelve days before surgery, at the last appointment with my breast surgeon before surgery, on Friday, May 29, at 4:30 p.m., I met with my doctor to go over last-minute details. I was now at peace with the decision of removing my right breast, although I have to admit I want to

ACTION ITEMS

ACTION ITEMS

use the word *resigned*; I'm a fighter! But I was at peace that this was the right decision for me.

Headed from the waiting area into the exam room, I sat down quietly to wait for the doctor. It was so silent, just dead quiet. Thoughts swirled in my head. It was maybe after a few minutes that I started to hear something. It was a very faint sound, maybe like music or talking, so I looked around the room thinking someone had left their cell phone. I checked mine, and it was not on. *Hm.* Where was this coming from? I then realized it was coming from my handbag!

Having watched too many movies, I started to think of the Matt Damon flick, *The Bourne Ultimatum,*[13] where he slips a cell phone in the journalist's pocket, and I thought, *Okay, maybe someone's cell somehow fell into my handbag—haha!* Okay, maybe a little too much time to think!

Anyway, I emptied my handbag, and there in my little purse I got in Paris, where I keep my iPod mini, the iPod was *somehow* turned on! And *really oddly,* it was playing an audio book that I had downloaded, gosh, at least many months earlier. While I had been meaning to listen to this audio book, I had never got the chance.

Strange, too, as I could have sworn the last item that I was listening to was a podcast by Dr. Charles Stanley. I also thought that even if I misremembered what I was listening to, I had a gazillion other iTunes, podcasts, and books on that iPod mini that could have come on. And still, how did it get turned on in the first place?

Yet it was playing this audio book, a memoir by Viktor E. Frankl, *Man's Search for Meaning,*[14] a very famous book. Frankl was an Austrian neurologist and psychiatrist who was a Holocaust survivor. In his book, he writes of how he overcame the

ACTION ITEMS

ACTION ITEMS

most dire of circumstances in a Nazi concentration camp and lived to tell about it. He is a founder of logotherapy, a form of existential analysis that has made tremendous contributions to the fields of psychology and philosophy.

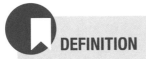

DEFINITION

LOGOTHERAPY[15]

A school of psychology and a philosophy based on the idea that we are strongly motivated to live purposefully and meaningfully, and that we find meaning in life as a result of responding authentically and humanely (i.e., meaningfully) to life's challenges.

This audio book recording, playing from my handbag, put in perspective what I was going through and the many challenges others in this world have faced and are facing right now that are far more difficult than my diagnosis with breast cancer.

Now I am not diminishing my challenges and difficulties as they are as real to me as yours are and will be for you, but I truly just sat there and . . . *thought.* I sat there quietly thinking and waiting in silence for what had to be another twenty minutes in this exam room on a Friday night as the very last patient, alone. Yes, I sat quietly and alone and thanked God for all the great blessings in my life and for that pinprick, that "sign" I believe and *know* He gave me. I prayed for those who have bigger mountains to move than mine. The door opened, and the doctor walked in.

I have since listened to Frankl's audio book. In closing this chapter, I want to share a passage from that book with you.

Action Items

Action Items

AN EXCERPT FROM DR. VIKTOR FRANKL'S BOOK
MAN'S SEARCH FOR MEANING

Between stimulus and response there is a space. In that space is our power to choose our response. In our response lies our growth and our freedom. Each man is questioned by life; and he can only answer to life by answering for his own life; to life he can only respond by being responsible. What is to give light must endure burning. Live as if you were living a second time, and as though you had acted wrongly the first time. Those who have a "why" to live can bear with almost any "how."[16]

"When we are no longer able
to change a situation, we are
challenged to change ourselves."

—*Viktor Frankl*[17]

Action Items

Action Items

NOTES

"There are two ways of spreading light; to be the candle or the mirror that reflects it."

— *Edith Wharton*[1]

Chapter Three
Breast Friends

I dedicate this chapter to all those *amazing* women and men who truly stepped it up and were there for me. They shared their experiences, helped guide my decisions, and, simply were just *there*. You all were lights in my life when I needed you the most—whether you knew how much of an impact you made or not.

I will never forget the powerful feelings of unconditional love, kindness, and warmth showered upon me. This book is my contribution, my way of paying it forward, to help those just diagnosed with breast cancer who, perhaps at this very moment, are just starting their very own journey.

You will take control of your diagnosis by doing your own research (based on science and facts), speaking with your doctors, talking with your breast friends, seeking spiritual guidance, and praying in your own way. Each person's diagnosis and journey are very different, and in this chapter I will share with you my and others' firsthand experiences in hopes they may be a guide for you.

I will share the "serendipitous" opportunities and people that came into my life at just the right time, helping me make my best decisions, from diagnosis to post-surgery care and recovery. So here we go.

After taking the initial tests and receiving the message on my cell phone from my breast surgeon confirming " . . . we've documented over 8 centimeters, and I really think you need a mastectomy, as I suspected . . ."—and once over the gasping phase!—I scheduled an appointment with the plastic surgeon. I then went on to schedule second and third appointments with additional breast and plastic surgeons. It was instinctive, really; there was no question I wanted numerous reviews of my tests and pathology and confirmation of my diagnosis and possible treatment options based on the diagnosis I was given.

MINI MENTION

Through my research I found exceptional healthcare providers as well as notable breast cancer centers of excellence around the United States. For obvious reasons—ease of travel time and expense—I decided to first look at those providers closest to my home, and you may want to do the same.

However, in perusing providers' websites from around the country, I came across many outstanding resources that were most helpful in both expected and unexpected ways. For instance, when I started to have tremendous anxiety about my impending surgery, I found, on the Johns Hopkins Kimmel Cancer Center website a forty-minute free yoga nidra video that helped to greatly relieve my anxiety, and to this day I still listen to it!

It was through reading and researching information (science and fact based) on many excellent provider websites that I would find the answers to one question and another would pop up. I also started to learn more about

ACTION ITEMS

ACTION ITEMS

meditation and integrative medicine. Here again, who knew that on my journey with breast cancer I'd be learning about meditation and integrative medicine?

While I ended up choosing to have my treatments and surgery locally, as I found the absolute best physicians for me were not far, if I'd had to travel, I would have. Your health is your number-one priority!

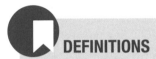

DEFINITIONS

YOGA NIDRA[2]

Yoga nidra is a guided meditation to induce full-body relaxation and deep rest. It helps quiet the overactive mind and brings it into a conscious, meditative state. Yoga nidra has been found to reduce symptoms of anxiety, posttraumatic stress disorder, chronic pain, and insomnia.

MEDITATION[3]

Meditation is a mind and body practice that has a long history of use for increasing calmness and physical relaxation, improving psychological balance, coping with illness, and enhancing overall health and wellbeing.

INTEGRATIVE MEDICINE[4]

Integrative medicine is a popular name for healthcare practices that traditionally have not been part of conventional medicine. Integrative medicine can help people with breast cancer, persistent pain, chronic fatigue, and

Action Items

Action Items

many other conditions better manage their symptoms and improve their quality of life by reducing fatigue, pain, and anxiety. Examples of common practices include:

- Acupuncture

- Animal-assisted therapy

- Aromatherapy

- Dietary supplements

- Massage therapy

- Music therapy

- Meditation

While I was going from doctor to doctor and office to office seeking medical guidance, I started to think, *I want to find other women who have already gone through this.* I wanted to hear the "real deal" and learn about their experiences firsthand.

I wanted to ask them questions like:

1. What was your diagnosis?

2. What type of procedures did you choose? Why?

3. What treatments did you decide to have? Why?

4. What was your overall journey like?

5. What, if anything, would you do differently?

Initially, I thought I knew no one with breast cancer! I had no friends, no family members, or anyone I could recall who'd

ACTION ITEMS

ACTION ITEMS

had breast cancer. So I thought, *Hm, how am I going to find people to speak with?* Chatting with a friend one day, she mentioned SHARE and Gilda's Club, two wonderful groups that support those with cancer. (*But I don't have cancer, do I? Yes, you will deny it!*) While they are exceptional organizations, I was in the midst of an outrageously busy work season and consumed with doctor appointments and taking tests; I just didn't have the time to check out new organizations or attend meetings. I thought, *Hm. How am I going to speed this up?*

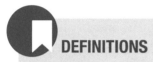

DEFINITIONS

SHARE[5]

SHARE is a national nonprofit that supports, educates, and empowers women affected by breast, ovarian, uterine, or metastatic breast cancer, with a special focus on medically underserved communities. Their mission is to connect these women with the unique support of survivors and peers, creating a community where no one has to face breast, ovarian, uterine, or metastatic breast cancer alone.

GILDA'S CLUB[6]

Gilda's Club NYC complements the medical component of cancer treatment by providing support and education for the cancer patient and their family to help them learn to live with cancer. Their program helps restore a sense of control, redefine hope, reduce stress and isolation, and educate participants to better manage their care during and after treatment.

ACTION ITEMS

ACTION ITEMS

Talking this over with gal pal Anita, she being my voice of reason, she said simply, "Arlene, just ask the doctor." I thought, *Why didn't I think about that?* So, as I said earlier, make sure to have a friend, family member, coworker, someone who will help think with and for you—you will be *overwhelmed*.

So at my next appointment with the breast surgeon I asked if she would connect me with other patients in her practice. (With a revolving door of breast cancer patients, should be a no-brainer, right?) She said no problem and that I should ask the surgical coordinator. Okay, I did. So, I'm waiting . . . and then my acknowledged type A personality kicked into high gear, and I called this woman a few more times with no response. Here's an example of a time where I think it is acceptable to be impatient! It was then I thought, *I'm not waiting on anyone.* And you won't want to either! I was like, *I'll find someone myself!* But where and whom?

With a fortunate stroke of serendipity unfolding, I had an encounter with Marie, a colleague, and as we were both grabbing a cup of coffee in our kitchen at work, I mentioned, "Hey, if you don't see me for a few weeks, it's okay. I'm having some breast stuff done. (I literally could not say the words *breast, cancer,* or *mastectomy* in any combination.) There was a brief pause, and she said, "I have a friend who had a double mastectomy. Would you like me to connect you both?" I said, "Yes, absolutely!"

Voila!

MY FIRST BREAST FRIEND

I left a message for Marie's friend Doris, and—and this is modus operandi (MO) with breast friends—she called me right back.

Doris shared that at thirty-nine (she's now fifty-seven), she was diagnosed with invasive lobule breast cancer and opted for a bilateral, or a double mastectomy. She went on to have breast

ACTION ITEMS

ACTION ITEMS

reconstruction and chose silicone breast implants. Doris was very happy with her choice. However, she did share that at one point in time years later her implant contracted but was quickly replaced, and overall, she was very happy. Following implant surgery, it's common for the breast to create a layer of scar tissue surrounding the implant known as a capsule. As time goes on, this capsule may tighten around the underlying implant, causing discomfort and distortion of the breast's appearance. Depending on the source you read and numerous variables such as type of implant (e.g., silicone or saline), contracture is reported in about 10 to 15 percent of women.[7] It is harmless in and of itself, but some women will seek revision surgery to correct the altered appearance.

Doris went on to say that the worst part for her was in the very beginning because to her, the implants did not feel completely natural. I asked why she had chosen silicone over saline breast implants; she replied silicone felt more natural. Most women I consulted and my doctors agreed, and I confirmed this through my research. Doris was so reassuring and a great comfort. She said my being proactive was great. That made me feel empowered.

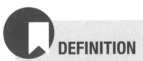

DEFINITION

CAPSULAR CONTRACTURE AND BREAST IMPLANTS[8]

Capsular contracture is a common complication of breast implant surgery that affects those who have augmentation or reconstruction. A capsule around a breast implant is a naturally occurring tissue that can be of benefit. If that capsule contracts or thickens, however, it can squeeze your implant. This contracture is what will cause pain, shifting, distortion, and hardening of the reconstructed breast.

Action Items

Action Items

Doris and I were on the phone for more than an hour. As our conversation came to an end, knowing my scheduled DIEP flap was just weeks away, I was still in search of someone who'd had that particular procedure. And with serendipity still unfolding, *voila!* Before we hung up the phone, she referred me to her friend June, who had had the DEIP flap procedure. And in less than twenty-four hours I had heard from June.

Today Doris is thriving. Here again, the breast friend MO: someone who didn't even know me at all and yet took the time to share unconditional support and inspiration.

MINI MENTION

As I was told my plastic surgeon "books well in advance" and that I needed to strategically book my surgery of a mastectomy after a busy work season (ending in May) but before the next (beginning in September), I scheduled the first of three surgeries for June 10 for the DIEP procedure. This was certainly not how I planned to use my summer vacation time or celebrate my upcoming fiftieth birthday but as one of my favorite lyrics goes in Lennon's "Beautiful Boy" song which contains the famous Allen Saunders quote "Life is what happens to you while you're busy making other plans."[9]

Since the surgeries for breast implants and DIEP flap require very different clinical teams and needs, I went ahead and initially scheduled the procedure. Like many women, I would come to embrace the main "selling point," which for me was that the DIEP flap uses a woman's own body tissue. So in my search to speak to others I greatly

ACTION ITEMS

ACTION ITEMS

wanted to find some women who had gone through the surgery. I was extremely glad to hear from June!

You too will seek out and find women who have, or had, your diagnosis!

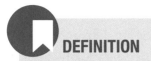

DEFINITION

BILATERAL OR DOUBLE MASTECTOMY[10]

If a mastectomy is done on both breasts, it is called a double (bilateral) mastectomy. When this is done, it is often a risk-reducing surgery for women at very high risk for breast cancer, such as those with a BRCA gene mutation or women with disease in both breasts.

MY SECOND BREAST FRIEND

June, at fifty-seven (now sixty-three), was diagnosed with DCIS in her right breast. *Well*, I thought, *that sounds familiar!* June chose to have a double mastectomy. This more aggressive treatment decision for the not-yet-cancer diagnosis of DCIS was chosen as June tested positive for the BRCA gene. And, as I would come to hear from other breast friends, she wanted to be *done with this*. She chose the DIEP flap because she wanted to use her own body tissue. This too was why I initially chose this procedure. June went on to share with me the real deal about this procedure and her experience.

She shared that while she was happy with the overall outcome of her surgery, the procedure lasted more than thirteen

ACTION ITEMS

ACTION ITEMS

hours since it was a double mastectomy. She spoke about the extensive healing process and that she had great difficulty sleeping. In addition to her chest area, she had an incision in her abdomen reaching from hip to hip. They give you that "bonus tummy tuck," she said, and I recalled that my plastic surgeon mentioned the same thing in our first meeting. They use your belly fat to build your new boob or, in June's case with a double mastectomy, two new ones. She said it was in her abdomen where she experienced the most pain and discomfort; however, she was up and walking around the very next day. And she went on to add that she had "nine Jackson-Pratt drains." (I'll define a JP drain shortly.) I thought, *A drain?* I hadn't read or heard about that. *Hm.* Ladies, get ready: here was yet another gasp! She went on to say she did not need radiation or chemotherapy.

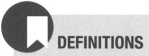

DEFINITIONS

RADIATION[11]

Radiation therapy is treatment with high-energy rays (or particles) that destroy cancer cells. Some women with breast cancer will need radiation in addition to other treatments.

CHEMOTHERAPY[12]

Chemotherapy is a drug treatment that uses powerful chemicals to kill fast-growing cells in your body. Chemotherapy is most often used to treat cancer since cancer cells grow and multiply much more quickly than most cells in the body.

ACTION ITEMS

ACTION ITEMS

June spent almost two hours with me on the phone. She went on to say that say was "thrilled with the results." And in true breast friend fashion, she was supportive in every way in sharing about her journey, all in hopes of making mine a little easier.

MINI MENTION

Let me stop and say another thing that will be key.

Ladies: everyone's recovery is different. While I was hats off to June for jumping out of bed the very next day, as doctors kept telling me we do need to get up and move, I was in tremendous pain. I was out of it. And while originally I told my work I'd be back in four weeks, I was back in six.

Be gentle with yourself. There is no rush. You must listen to *your* body and take the time to heal at *your* pace. As I've said throughout this book, while we will hear from our doctors and speak with our breast friends and uncover much information during our research on "what to expect-know and do," we then must weigh our options and ultimately do what is best for us!

DEFINITIONS

BRCA GENE[13]

"BRCA" is an abbreviation for "BReast CAncer gene." BRCA1 and BRCA2 are two different genes that have been found to impact a person's chances of developing breast cancer. Every human has both the BRCA1 and

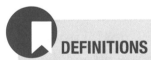

Action Items

Action Items

BRCA2 genes. Despite what their names might suggest, BRCA genes do not cause breast cancer. In fact, these genes normally play a big role in preventing breast cancer. They help repair DNA breaks that can lead to cancer and the uncontrolled growth of tumors. Because of this, the BRCA genes are known as tumor suppressor genes. However, in some people these tumor suppression genes do not work properly. When a gene becomes altered or broken, it doesn't function correctly. This is called a gene mutation.

JACKSON-PRATT (JP) DRAIN[14]

This is a closed–suction medical device commonly used as a postoperative drain for collecting bodily fluids from surgical sites. The drain itself is inside the body. It is made of Teflon and has multiple drainage holes. The drain is connected to clear plastic tubing, which is usually sutured to the skin at the point it leaves the skin. The tubing connects to a bulb reservoir. The bulb, when squeezed empty, applies constant suction to the drain and pulls the fluid out of the body. The drain is removed when excess fluid has stopped draining from the body. Removal does not usually require an anesthetic. The purpose of a drain is to prevent fluid (blood or other) buildup in a closed ("dead") space, which may cause either disruption of the wound and the healing process or become an infected abscess—with either scenario possibly requiring a formal drainage/repair procedure (and possibly another trip to the operating room). If the drainage tubing becomes clogged or otherwise clotted off, the benefits from drainage are not realized.

Action Items

Action Items

A NEW GROUP OF FRIENDS, BREAST FRIENDS

Yes! I was introduced to many new breast friends, and frankly, I was not prepared to find the *staggeringly large numbers* of women who had, have, or know of someone close to them—like a mom, sister, sister-in-law, aunt, cousin, or friend—with breast cancer!

It was like a snowball effect. I spoke with one woman one day and she suggested, "Hey, why don't you speak with . . . ?" and so on and so on. From knowing not one person with breast cancer, it was now like almost everyone I spoke with either had or knew of someone with breast cancer. Truly, it was crazy. I thought breast cancer was well under control! All the "pink" out there, all the walks, the extensive research and fundraising to cure breast cancer. I honestly had *no idea* it was so commonplace.

At this point that I realized I had accumulated a mountain of notes—aka my 63,000 words—and I was becoming overwhelmed with meeting so many new breast friends. I thought, *How am I going to keep track of the numerous phone numbers, emails, and valuable notes?* At first I thought I'd just add them to my general friends group in Outlook, but then I realized *they are special friends.* And in that moment the words *breast friends* popped in my mind, which is how I have come to define them: women—*and men*—who instinctively knew the journey I was about to embark on and were there to help! I started a new group called "Breast Friends."

 MINI MENTION

While I had many amazing people supporting me, be ready to experience some who may let you down. While

ACTION ITEMS

ACTION ITEMS

there were countless strangers there to lift me up and support me, there were those I expected to count on who were either not there at all or not as fully committed to helping as I would have liked.

We all have our own capacity to handle life's curveballs, and I tend to think that their avoidance, in whatever manner, or lack of support, could have been *their* coping mechanism.

As it was down to that very last doctor's appointment as I wrestled with the reality of a mastectomy, my friends and family did too! Perhaps they just couldn't imagine this for themselves. And perhaps they just couldn't believe that someone who looked healthy and so full of life was not well. *And I couldn't either.*

MY THIRD BREAST FRIEND

So as serendipity would have it, in late May, I had a doctor's appointment and I was the next-to-last patient. Sitting there, I overheard a patient say, "Okay, I'll call you about the tattoo." Having done my research, I knew what she was referring to and quickly assessed that she had already likely had a mastectomy. So without going completely type A on her and cornering her in the doctor's office, I thought, *How am I going to get her attention in the hope she will talk with me?* As she walked past, I let out a loud sigh and said, "Ahhh, gosh, life is crazy," hoping she'd stop to chat. And she did. *Voila!*

She introduced herself as Dana. We sat together for about twenty minutes, and she shared that a year earlier, at age

Action Items

Action Items

fifty-one, she'd had a double mastectomy. And twenty years earlier, she'd had ovarian cancer. While she tested negative for the BRCA gene, she opted for a double mastectomy to ensure she never has to deal with this again—a comment, by the way, I heard frequently. She went on to say she had the DIEP breast reconstruction procedure. *Voila!* One more breast friend with the procedure I was going to have. I asked her why she chose that procedure. Like me, she also wanted her own flesh as part of her reconstruction. I also asked her about the tattoo and that process and her experience.

She went on to share that she was extremely happy with the results—although she did develop necrosis right after surgery. Here I recalled the plastic surgeon mentioning in our first meeting the possibility of necrosis as very minimal at 1 to 2 percent. Dana sarcastically said to me that she was "the lucky 1 percent." She explained they took the steps to correct it, which included another surgery, and a year later she was perfectly happy with her results. As Doris also shared, Dana said the worst and most painful part was the abdominal incision. She also shared she decided to take Tamoxifen.

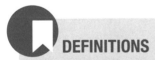

DEFINITIONS

NECROSIS[15]

This is death of body tissue and occurs when there is not enough blood flowing to the tissue whether from injury, radiation, or chemicals. Necrosis is not reversible. When substantial areas of tissue die due to a lack of blood supply, the condition is called gangrene.

Action Items

Action Items

GANGRENE[16]

Gangrene is the death of tissue in part of the body. Gangrene happens when a body part loses its blood supply. This may happen from injury, an infection, or other causes.

TAMOXIFEN[17]

Tamoxifen is the oldest and most-prescribed selective estrogen receptor modulator (SERM). Tamoxifen is approved by the U.S. Food and Drug Administration (FDA) to treat women and men diagnosed with hormone-receptor-positive, early-stage breast cancer after surgery (or possibly chemotherapy and radiation) to reduce the risk of the cancer coming back.

BREAST TATTOO[18]

3D nipple tattoos are real tattoos applied with needles that insert pigment into the skin. An experienced nipple tattoo artist can create an amazingly realistic image of a nipple that appears to have physical dimension but is really flat to the touch. In recent years, a growing number of people have been opting for 3D nipple tattoos instead of nipple reconstruction surgery. Also, plastic surgeons often recommend 3D nipple tattoos instead of nipple reconstruction surgery. Nipple tattooing can also be done to enhance the results of nipple reconstruction surgery.

After speaking with my three new breast friends Doris, June, and Dana, I started to get more of an understanding about what

ACTION ITEMS

ACTION ITEMS

I was in for having a mastectomy and what I was to expect on my journey ahead.

Also, after hearing about June's and Dana's experiences with the DIEP procedure, I was having great reservations about moving forward with that surgery. I recalled the plastic surgeon saying there was only a 1 to 2 percent chance of necrosis, but out of the two breast friends I met who'd had the DIEP procedure, one developed necrosis! That's 50 percent! *Just sayin'.* It was also around this time that my breast surgeon directed me to take a CT angiogram. I thought, *Hm, that's the first I'm hearing of that test.* Prepare; a gasp is coming!

Then I started to think about the length of the surgery and being under anesthesia for more than four to six hours. Being in great health most of my life, I never really had a major surgery other than the removal of my tonsils as a small child, and my appendix was removed about fifteen years ago, but that was a minimally invasive laparoscopic surgery. Being under anesthesia for that amount of time completely freaked me out. I was in fear of not waking up! Then I started to read about anesthesia and thought, *Who's in charge of dispensing that?* (More on that later.) I thought it would be nice to have a bonus tummy tuck, but the painful recovery and extensive incision and scarring on my abdomen from hip to hip—not to mention the painful recovery of my chest—greatly concerned me.

And as if all that wasn't enough to think about, I was reading up on the CT angiogram and found it basically tests for blood flow, and I was like, *Blood flow? For what?!* They were going to take veins and blood vessels that had been settled down in my abdomen for all my life and move them north to my chest! All to build my new breast! Yikes!

Action Items

Action Items

DEFINITIONS

CT ANGIOGRAM[19]

This is a special type of CT scan that evaluates the blood flow in the abdomen to determine if the required blood vessels are intact and able to be used for DIEP flap reconstruction. It can also provide a "road map" for the surgeon and help locate the larger blood vessels (perforators).

An angiogram is an imaging test that uses X-rays to look at the patient's blood vessels. An abdominal angiogram looks at the blood vessels in your abdomen. It may be used to check blood flow to the organs of the abdomen such as the liver and spleen. It may also be used as a guide in the placement of medicine or other materials to treat cancer or bleeding in the abdomen. *Fluoroscopy* is often used during an abdominal angiogram. This is a kind of X-ray "movie" with continuous X-rays showing the provider real-time images of the test procedure.

Contrast dye is used to cause the blood vessels to appear solid on the X-ray image. This lets the radiologist see the blood vessels more clearly. Dye is injected into specific blood vessels to look at a certain area of blood flow more closely. For an abdominal angiogram, a catheter (small tube) is placed into a large artery in your groin and then placed into the specific artery of interest. Contrast is injected through this tube. Next, the radiologist takes a series of X-ray pictures. These images show the blood flow in the abdomen. You may also have a CT (computed tomography) scan or MRI (magnetic resonance imaging) scan with your angiogram.

ACTION ITEMS

ACTION ITEMS

ANESTHESIOLOGIST[20]

An anesthesiologist is a doctor (MD or DO) who practices anesthesia. Anesthesiologists are physicians specializing in perioperative care, developing anesthetic plans, and the administration of anesthetics.

MINI MENTION

You may find yourself wondering what a tattoo could possibly have to do with breast cancer. Here again was another unexpected find on my journey! So here we go: we are going to talk about nipples and tattoos!

While not everyone opts for breast reconstruction, I did. I chose a breast implant and, for me, it entailed three surgical procedures. The first was when they did the mastectomy and put in a tissue expander; the second came when they removed the tissue expander and put in the actual implant in my right breast so it was all even. And the third was when they created a nipple. The tattoo is the fourth or final step one can choose—or not—in putting yourself back together.

When you have a mastectomy you may lose your nipple and the areola around it. Why? The cancer and disease may have spread to that area. So you also may find yourself having to make the decision of whether to have your nipple removed.

So while doctors agreed that with the extensive amount of DCIS a mastectomy is optimal, I had two doctors with

Action Items

Action Items

varying opinions on removing my nipple. One doctor said I could leave it and the other, who ended up being my surgeon, said, "You should remove it." However, she could do a biopsy during surgery to identify whether there were abnormal cells lurking in the nipple. But she noted that a biopsy pulls a small sampling of tissue and, even if it was negative, that wouldn't necessarily mean there weren't bad cells in there somewhere. Well, that I knew firsthand, as remember, both earlier breast needle biopsies missed the Invasive cancer cells lurking! Just sayin'!

This was still a most difficult decision as I wanted to keep as many body parts as possible, and I know you will too, but then I thought, in the same moment, what happens if the disease is missed? Would this all be for nothing? While usually pretty good at making decisions, I simply did not know what to do. As I thought about whether to keep the nipple or not, my gal pal Hallia popped into my mind. I called her immediately. In just the space of a brief call and a question, she simply asked, "Arlene! Why would you leave an old part on a new car?" That was it. My decision was made. The nipple was going! And thus, on my third surgery, I had nipple reconstruction.

So back to the tattoo! After all your surgery is completed and after months of healing, you are eligible to get a tattoo. Okay, but who does breast tattoos?! While I continued to speak with breast friends, I noticed a trend emerging. Almost all women who had chosen to color the nipple and create a new areola—aka a breast tattoo—had a doctor do this. Everyone I spoke with was unhappy with this outcome.

ACTION ITEMS

ACTION ITEMS

The responses ranged from "it wasn't the right size and didn't match" to "the color was off" to "it faded quickly." Now I don't have any tattoos but thought, *Why would you go to a medical doctor for a tattoo?* I certainly wouldn't go to a tattoo artist for breast surgery, right? Just sayin'!

Thus, after much research on the internet, I found an amazing artist known for his and his team's work in helping women who have had mastectomies put themselves back together. Vinnie Myers's tattoo shop is located in Finksburg, Maryland.[21] They are *amazing*. And me and gal pal Anita were off to get me a breast tattoo!

More on this later, but since I know you must be wondering what that process can be like, here are a few mentions on what to expect: Before going to Vinnie's you will need to send photos of both breasts before you get to your appointment; they need to be assessed. They will then contact you with results and make an appointment. When you arrive at Vinnie's, you will be asked to fill out paperwork. Then you'll go into a room and sit in the artist chair with breasts bared: *cringe*. Trent, who worked with me, then matched the color closest to my other areola. I guess in the case of a double mastectomy, you choose your own areola color! By the way, while most of my breast was numb from surgery, part was not, and it does hurt!

And yes, this was yet another unexpected experience in my journey with breast cancer—I know, at forty-nine (okay, fifty!) I have my first tattoo on my breast! Another *who knew* kind of moment!

Action Items

Action Items

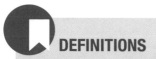

DEFINITIONS

BREAST RECONSTRUCTION USING A TISSUE EXPANDER AND IMPLANT[22]

After your breast surgeon completes the mastectomy, if you have an implant-based breast reconstruction surgery, your plastic surgeon may use a tissue expander. In this type of reconstruction, your plastic surgeon will make a pocket under a large muscle (the pectoralis) in your chest and place a tissue expander in that space. A tissue expander is an empty breast implant that will be filled with normal saline over six to eight weeks. This process slowly stretches your skin and pectoralis muscle. When the expander reaches the size your surgeon and you agree on, they stop the expansion process. About four to eight weeks after the tissue expansion is finished, you will have a second surgery to remove the tissue expander and insert the permanent breast implant. If you will be having chemotherapy or radiation therapy, your doctor will tell you when your implant will be placed.

NIPPLE RECONSTRUCTION[23]

If you decide to have nipple reconstruction, you may have that done about two to four months after the permanent breast implant is placed. Nipple reconstruction surgery is usually an outpatient procedure that uses skin from the area of the breast where the nipple will be located to form a new nipple. Later, the reconstructed nipple may be tattooed to add color and to create the areola.

Action Items

Action Items

MY FOURTH BREAST FRIEND

Here again came another serendipitous opportunity to connect with another breast friend. I recalled an outstanding keynote speaker I had met months earlier in January at the annual Alliance for Continuing Education in the Health Professions (ACEhp) healthcare conference I attended. This year it was held in Dallas, Texas. She spoke so eloquently about her journey with breast cancer and the difficulties patients encounter as we navigate through the treacherous terrain of our already-overburdened health systems.

As I recalled her talk, I realized she had addressed some of the very issues I was now experiencing as a patient. Instead of calling to hire her to speak at one of my educational conferences, I'd be seeking her guidance on *my* diagnosis. Another *who knew?* moment!

I called the conference organizer and didn't have to say much more than, "Hey, Ales. I need contact information for . . . ." She quickly shared Laura's email. Now late April, I reached out to her. Laura, a busy career woman, and not knowing me at all, in true breast friend fashion, reached out immediately to someone who just happened to see her speak at a conference months before some fifteen hundred miles away!

 MINI MENTION

Where there is a will there is a way! Do not hesitate to reach out to others for help. Do not be embarrassed, or if you are, okay, take a moment, relish in it, then as my gal pal Anita would say, "Get over it!" You need to. Be persistent. Ask questions—a lot of them! It is okay. *We are in this together!*

ACTION ITEMS

ACTION ITEMS

Laura addressed issues I was too embarrassed to discuss and frankly didn't even think to ask. As I reflect back, in some unconscious way, I was afraid to hear the answers. Yet intuitively, with eloquence and grace, she presented those awkward issues and questions and answered them all for me, someone she didn't even know—other than I was someone just diagnosed with breast cancer. I was overwhelmed by her sincere and complete openness to share her story as I now entered the "sisterhood." She was someone who knew firsthand what lay ahead for me.

Like me, Laura was diagnosed with DCIS of the right breast, tested negative for the BRCA gene, and chose to have a mastectomy of only her right breast. She opted for an implant, silicone. She took Tamoxifen for five years. She is doing fantastic and thriving today! Laura was monumental in helping me make several decisions. She made herself completely available for the entire first year of my journey. We went on to speak several times on the phone, via emails, and through texts. Six years later, Laura and I are still in touch. She *never* wavered and always kept herself available to me. Laura, thank you!

BREAST FRIENDS FIVE AND SIX AND MAKING FINAL DECISIONS

Yes! Each new breast friend brought a new perspective to my journey. I went from not knowing anyone with breast cancer to, within weeks, hearing from so many women who shared their stories openly and lovingly. Finally, I felt like it was now coming together from doing my research, hearing from those amazing breast friends, getting several doctors' opinions, and praying and seeking spiritual guidance. I was well informed to be able to make the best decisions for myriad questions and procedures I had to address—and finalize.

Action Items

Action Items

However, I still had an unidentifiable, haunting, unsettled feeling that *something was still missing*, but I couldn't put my finger on it. But it was my next serendipitous yet perfectly timed encounters with two unexpected new breast friends— one who happened to be a doctor from California and one whom I had been working with for three years—that made a new, huge impact. These two would help me identify that *still missing* feeling.

While joking with friends that there's no good time for surgery, as life as you know it comes to an abrupt halt when you are *just diagnosed*, the timing was perfect as my surgery came at the tail end of a busy work season.

A THORACIC SURGEON

Earlier on, in mid-March, I managed an annual thoracic chest medicine conference now going into its third year. I felt privileged having had the opportunity to work through the years with an outstanding lead surgeon, his course directors, and their talented faculty. This conference was exactly around the time I got that call on the Long Island Rail Road saying my MRI lit up and that I needed to take those three additional tests, one being a CT chest scan.

I never could have imagined that Dr. Richard Lazzaro, a thoracic surgeon I had been working with for three years, would be pivotal in some of the decisions I would now make in my journey with breast cancer. Yes! Another *who knew?* kind of moment.

Now late April, with myriad tests behind me and being told a mastectomy may be imminent, a thought popped in my mind. *Hm, while the CT chest scan came back with "There is no abnormality to account for the small focus of signal abnormality on the right lung," why don't I reach out to Dr. Lazzaro?*

Action Items

Action Items

While I didn't have a thoracic issue, I had grown very fond of working with him and thought I'd like to get an appointment and get his opinion. But why would a thoracic surgeon meet with me about a breast cancer diagnosis? But I did have a CT scan he could review. *Hm . . . voila!* So I called his office.

Now late May, just fourteen days before my scheduled surgery, he met with me for more than an hour. I never gave up hoping for someone, anyone, to say, "You don't have to have a mastectomy." He did not say those words either. He did, however, review with me my scans, films, and prior reports. He went on to share he was familiar with DCIS. I had come to trust his opinion and felt more at peace speaking with him, and he gave me confidence in what I needed to do. And he reconfirmed that I was in the best of hands with my doctors. While I loved my breast surgeon—she is amazing—I really didn't know her except for meeting her once or twice, and I was initially extremely apprehensive.

So as our time was coming to an end and I was furiously taking notes, I scribbled things down quickly when he said, "Embrace the moment and let fear go. Not letting go holds us back." This resonated strongly with me. As we were wrapping up our time together, I asked him one last question. He shared, paraphrasing him, the goals of surgery are:

1. Be okay.

2. Get out the cancer.

3. Put it all back together in the least invasive way.

It was after this meeting I knew what I needed to do as he helped me to find the answers already within me. He was very inspirational.

ACTION ITEMS

ACTION ITEMS

A WEST COAST DOCTOR

Now late May and ironically at my very last conference, eleven days before surgery I met Dr. Ricki Pollycove. While this conference was focused specifically on women's heart health, it also focused on women's health in general and had an outstanding faculty. It was at the faculty dinner hosted the night before, when everyone introduced themselves, that one doctor stood out to me: Dr. Ricki Pollycove. So that night I got home and researched her and found she had an outstanding national reputation as a leader in the promotion of women's wellness, patient empowerment, breast health, and integrative medicine. Breast health! Integrative medicine! Really! I had to speak with her! In some way I was still holding out, still hoping someone, anyone, would tell me something different and say, "Arlene, you do not need a mastectomy to remove your right breast!" And she did not say those words either.

Down to the wire I reached out to Dr. Pollycove, and in that fabulous breast friend style, in less than twenty-four hours she emailed me a lovely and inspirational note. She noted, in part, "Take good care of the sisterhood." As I had missed she was based on the West Coast and we were scheduling time to talk on the phone, she went on to say, "I'll keep EDT in mind!" Can you imagine? This busy, nationally renowned doctor from across the country, who doesn't know me at all, who responds to my email immediately and calls the very next day, is thinking about me and considerate of my time zone. Who are these people? They are *amazing* breast friends. And you too will have them right alongside you on your journey!

We spoke on the phone for more than forty-five minutes. I furiously took notes. She was such an inspiration. You know how some people just have that special "it" factor? Well, she was

Action Items

Action Items

overflowing with "it"! She said I was "highly intuitive." This made me feel empowered and proud that I had done the best I could on my journey to date, that I was a fighter, and that I was on top of my diagnosis. She shared some thoughts from my diagnosis to possible treatments and procedures. At one point during our conversation, I asked her about the DIEP procedure and what she thought. However, I had become accustomed to hearing this phrase from literally every single doctor. To paraphrase: "I can't give you my opinion. You'll have to make that decision on your own." It was like a mantra I heard from office to office, so while I asked, I wasn't really expecting her to answer. But even before I finished my sentence she replied, "Oh no. No, I will tell you exactly what I think." I was overwhelmed with gratitude and thankful for her directness and honesty. I was exhausted at this point. I was thought out! I was done. I now knew what I had to do. I felt complete.

That *something missing* feeling was no more!

THE UNIVERSE UNFOLDING AS IT SHOULD (*DESIDERATA*)[24]

I'm always amazed how the universe works. Just the right people and opportunities show up and come into my life, delivering what I may need at exactly the right moment . . . it's fascinating! And they will for you—guaranteed. You just have to be open, watching, and expecting.

The book is peppered with the words *choice* and *chance*. We always have choices, and I believe nothing is simply by chance. We can in great part create our own destiny. As I said in the preface, while I may be destined to live to be 101, if I choose to walk in front of a bus, I very well may not live to be 101.

I have found the little serendipitous events that occur in any one day in life to be exciting, and I try my best to always be

ACTION ITEMS

ACTION ITEMS

aware and open to receiving them. I plan for them by doing my best to cut through the noise of the day and stay open. It's in the stillness and quietness of these moments when we surrender ourselves that the greatest gifts and surprises tend to come our way!

And so it was with these last two completely unexpected breast friends that I met along my journey, at the very last moment—at peace (the best I could find while removing a body part of forty-nine years—almost fifty), I knew, deep down, what I needed to do—I was getting a mastectomy. I changed the surgery—literally ten days prior—from DIEP procedure to a breast implant. My surgery was scheduled for Wednesday, June 10, 2015.

"Embrace the moment and let fear go. Not letting go holds us back."

—*Richard Lazzaro, MD*

Action Items

Action Items

NOTES

NOTES

"A mind that is stretched by a new experience can never go back to its old dimensions."

—*Oliver Wendell Holmes, Jr.*

Part Two
Why, When, How
Breast Cancer

"Let us not look back in anger, nor forward in fear, but around in awareness."

—*James Thurber*[1]

Chapter Four
Breast Cancer Is a Disease That Does Not Discriminate

A s I started my journey through extensive conversations, it became apparent breast cancer has no borders; it does not discriminate by age or gender; by race, social, or financial status; by celebrity; or by how high you have climbed the career ladder. And while both incidence and mortality have dropped over the last two decades[2] and there have been increases in the five- and ten-year survival rates, breast cancer is still quite prevalent and affects extraordinarily large numbers of individuals within our population. Paradoxically, despite the rate of incidence dropping since 1999, due to the growing and aging total population, the total number of cases annually has grown.

When I was reviewing and editing this chapter, I thought, *What is the purpose of including it? How is this chapter going to help* you *on your journey, having been just diagnosed with breast cancer?*

Then the answer quickly came to me: comfort in knowing that you are not alone. This chapter shows the evolution, from that first conversation, from that first time you open up and talk to someone, *anyone*, about being just diagnosed, that you will quickly realize, as I did, that there is a network of breast cancer survivors right in the midst of your circle of friends, family, and colleagues. And while I initially felt so alone, isolated, and as though I was the only one with breast cancer, as I started to open up and speak with others, there was an emerging trend: almost everyone I spoke with had a story about someone they knew with breast cancer—*almost everyone.*

BREAST CANCER DOES NOT DISCRIMINATE BY GENDER, AGE, RACE

As vice president of communications in my local political club, I made a point during the politically quieter summer months to connect with our board members. In August, just eight weeks after my mastectomy, I called Don, a longtime board member. I wanted to see how his summer was going and talk about the upcoming (2016) presidential election and how our club would ramp up for September political events. When we made connections and I asked how he was, he immediately said, "Not so well." While not expecting this response, I said, "What's going on?"

Don shared he had just been diagnosed with breast cancer. A huge lump was found in his right breast. It was on this call, and for the first time, that I chose to publicly share my very recent journey with Don. I wanted to comfort him and let him know he was not alone. As many had done for me, I listened attentively to his story and wanted to make sure he was on the right track with tests, treatments, and getting a second opinion. Thinking back, it was at that exact moment that I crossed over and become a breast friend to someone else—paying it forward.

Action Items

Action Items

He was in his seventies and African-American. Breast cancer does not discriminate by gender, age, or race.

MINI MENTION

And as I was initially sharing my story with two members of my club leadership in late May, telling them I was going to be less active in the club for a few weeks after surgery, there was a brief, silent pause. Then my club president, now in her sixties, shared that in her thirties she had breast cancer, chose to have a mastectomy, and did not opt for reconstruction. Breast cancer affects even young women.

BREAST CANCER DOES NOT DISCRIMINATE BY AGE, CELEBRITY, GENDER

As I prepared to let my colleagues, clients, and consultants know that I would be out of work for about four to six weeks (it ended up being six), I was having a more personal conversation with my marketing consultant, Marie, who had become a friend. When I shared my news with her, there was that brief, silent pause I had come to know all too well. She then shared with me her husband's cousin recently tested positive for the BRCA gene and chose to have a double mastectomy and earlier on, in her years, she had to remove her ovaries. Like most women I heard from, Marie said, this woman wanted to be done with this. Marie told me another friend of hers, in her thirties, recently tested positive for the BRCA gene and also chose to have a double mastectomy and hysterectomy.

Action Items

Action Items

When I went back to work in late August, Marie and I reconnected as I ramped up for fall programs. Catching up on the phone one day, I shared Don's story and how I never knew men could have breast cancer. She went on to tell me that her husband, a big fan of the rock band KISS, shared the band's former drummer, Peter Criss, was diagnosed with breast cancer. Wow! I grew up listening to KISS. Who knew? So I looked it up, and in 2007, Criss noticed a painful lump in his chest while working out and, because his wife was battling another form of cancer at the time, he didn't hesitate to get it checked out. In February 2008, doctors removed what they believed was a harmless nodule from Criss's chest, but tests revealed that nodule was breast cancer. Another surgery, in March 2008, removed the cancer, and thankfully the cancer had not spread and Criss didn't need to undergo chemotherapy. That same year, as reported by *Rolling Stone* magazine and as a guest on CNN, Criss shared his story openly to bring awareness to National Breast Cancer Month. He (like me) talked about his scare and that he didn't even know men could get breast cancer until he was diagnosed. He went on to say, "So many people must die from this. . . . Somebody has to step up to the plate and say something to get them aware of how dangerous this is. Lots of men die: They wait, they don't go in, they put it off."[3] Thankfully, Criss treated the disease before it could spread and is now cancer-free.

BREAST CANCER DOES NOT DISCRIMINATE BY BORDERS OR HOW HIGH YOU'VE CLIMBED THE CORPORATE LADDER

Post-surgery, in late July, sharing my news for the first time with my BFF and great friend Colton in Toronto, Canada, once again I was met with that brief, silent pause. He quickly

ACTION ITEMS

ACTION ITEMS

shared his brother-in-law's sister, now in her mid-forties, had been just diagnosed with Stage 4 breast cancer and that she was "barely hanging on." He said she'd had signs but did not bother to go to the doctors and follow up. Hear this: *We never think "it" will happen to us.* If you feel something is not right, it may very well not be. Go to the doctor and get it checked out. If it's nothing great but it is something, wouldn't you rather know about it and have caught it early on? *Yes! I knew you'd agree!* Colton also said a friend of his who had just turned fifty passed away after battling breast cancer for ten years. She had been a busy and successful career woman in the United States who had recently moved back to Toronto to be with her family. Devastating.

MINI MENTION

Ladies, *and men*, while I hope this is starting to resonate clearly through this book, we must be aware! *We must listen to our bodies!* Then take action. There were many women I spoke with who had signs and (like me) chose to take action and men, like Peter Criss, who went to their doctors and thwarted the worst. Then there are those who choose to do nothing, like my BFF's sister-in-law; she let it go. She ignored the signs until it was too late.

A good friend of mine was visiting from Arizona in late August, and she was aware of my upcoming surgery in June; we finally had a chance to catch up in person. She shared that a wonderful friend of hers had passed away a year earlier after having been diagnosed with breast

Action Items

Action Items

cancer. Her friend chose to not take action; a year later the cancer metastasized to her brain and took her life.

Why do some choose to take action and others do not? Fear? Perception—not wanting to lose a breast as they may feel "less" a woman? Embarrassment? Do they think if they ignore it, it will just go away? Whatever the reason, they make their choices, and you will too. We have choices. While I would never judge an individual's decision as to what they think is the best course for their life, I feel compelled to note we are not our breasts. And I ask, *is that breast worth possibly giving up your life for?* I understand society may put a lot of pressure on us as women to look a certain way, but we must not place that pressure on ourselves. And by the way, with the advancements of breast reconstruction surgery, they can look great! (More on this in chapter seven)

We must be confident in the inherent value we give back to society each and every day as a mom, sister, daughter, wife, friend, or colleague. We must not be judged or, worst of all, judge ourselves by our breasts or the size of them. My political club president chose not to do breast reconstruction; I did. For each of us, that was the best decision.

So as I struggled to decide what I should do (and you will likely too)—whether to not have a mastectomy and keep getting breast biopsies every six months in the hopes the DCIS wouldn't spread or turn into "real" cancer, or just have the mastectomy and be rid of the disease—the question that kept

Action Items

Action Items

nagging at my gut may be the one nagging at you. *How much treatment is too much, and how much is not enough?*

While I'll address this directly in chapter eight, let me say here that after my mastectomy in June an article came out in *Time* magazine[4] in October 2015. I still have that issue, and on the cover a woman is holding her breast and the caption says, "What if I do nothing?" Well, as I read the article, I immediately had that gut-wrenching, sinking, sickening feeling in my stomach and thought, *My God, should I not have removed my breast?* Did I do too much? But then, immediately, in nearly the same split-second as I was having that thought, I also thought, *No,* as, remember, it wasn't until after the surgery that they found invasive cancer and staged my breast cancer as Stage 1A. I absolutely made the right choice.

You will research your diagnosis, speak with your breast friends, seek your doctors' guidance, get second opinions, review your tests and pathology, listen to your gut, and ultimately you will make the most informed decision for you! It was based on all those things that I chose to have that mastectomy and without knowing that both those breast biopsies missed the invasive cancer already in my body! Not knowing the DCIS had already turned into invasive cancer, I chose to have that mastectomy. And thank God I did. You too will choose the best for you. It will be okay. Choose wisely.

BREAST CANCER DOES NOT DISCRIMINATE BY BORDERS

Years back a good friend of mine (still is today) from the New York Stock Exchange introduced me to her friend Christiane who lives in Paris, France. Ever since that first introduction, when we picnicked in Riverside Park on Manhattan's Upper West Side, we have traded apartments for a few weeks a year,

ACTION ITEMS

ACTION ITEMS

where I'm in her fabulous flat waking up and falling asleep with an amazing view of the Eiffel Tower, and she loves the Upper West Side. Christiane is a wonderful person and friend. This year while she was in town, I shared my news with her. And after that, yes . . . brief, silent pause, which I have come to know all too well. Christiane, who at this point had known me for more than ten years, went on to tell me for the first time that she'd had breast cancer and four surgeries in the past two years. I never knew. We never talked about it. Breast cancer does not discriminate by geography.

MINI MENTION

While I was embarrassed, I want you to learn from my experience and know you *do not* have to be afraid or embarrassed to talk about your diagnosis. Can you imagine? Christiane and I knew each other for more than ten years and never talked about it.

I hope you are now seeing how my awareness about the prevalence of breast cancer evolved from that first conversation on. Truly, it still blows my mind as the greatest irony is that while I thought I knew no one with breast cancer, it was literally all around me.

I thought, *How could I have been so ignorant of the staggering numbers of women and men with breast cancer? Hm.* For, other than the fanfare in October deemed Breast Cancer Awareness Month in the United States, it is a silent and lonely disease eleven months of the rest of the year. I felt alone in the beginning. I didn't know how to start that first conversation, or whom to start it with, or where to

Action Items

Action Items

start searching for that first breast friend—until I started to just simply open up and share.

Do not be afraid or embarrassed to share your story first. While this is a very intimately placed disease, it is cancer. And from grabbing that cup of coffee at work and Marie walking up, from that first conversation when she introduced me to Doris who then introduced me to June, well, the floodgates were opened!

Open up to a close friend or maybe someone more removed! Anyway you choose to, I promise you, those breast friends are right there in your circle. And they are just waiting to help!

BREAST CANCER DOES NOT DISCRIMINATE BY CELEBRITY OR FINANCIAL STATUS

Also near the time of my diagnosis, several high-profile celebrity cases of breast cancer were reported like Rita Wilson—American actress, singer, songwriter, producer, and married to actor Tom Hanks. In April of that year, she underwent a double mastectomy and reconstructive surgery[5] at age fifty-eight. Her diagnosis almost missed until, she said, a friend who had had breast cancer suggested she get a second opinion on her pathology, and as I did and you hopefully will too, she followed her gut and got that second opinion. A different pathologist found invasive lobular carcinoma, and her diagnosis was confirmed. Breast cancer does not discriminate by celebrity or financial status. Moreover, even a person with considerable wealth and access to the best doctors can face this misdiagnosis. That's why you too must take charge by asking questions and doing your own science-based research.

Action Items

Action Items

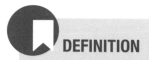

DEFINITION

LOBULAR CARCINOMA IN SITU (LCIS)[6]

This is an area (or areas) of abnormal cell growth that increases a person's risk of developing invasive breast cancer later in life. Lobular means that the abnormal cells start growing in the lobules, the milk-producing glands at the end of breast ducts. Carcinoma refers to any cancer that begins in the skin or other tissues that cover internal organs, such as breast tissue. In situ, or "in its original place," means that the abnormal growth remains inside the lobule and does not spread to surrounding tissues. People diagnosed with LCIS tend to have more than one lobule affected. The breast contains about fifteen to twenty lobules.

Despite the fact that its name includes the term *carcinoma*, LCIS is not a true breast cancer. Rather, LCIS is an indication that a person is at higher-than-average risk for getting breast cancer at some point in the future. For this reason, some experts prefer the term *lobular neoplasia* instead of *lobular carcinoma*. A neoplasia is a collection of abnormal cells.

LCIS is viewed as an uncommon condition, but we don't know exactly how many people are affected. That's because LCIS does not cause symptoms and usually does not show up on a mammogram. It tends to be diagnosed through a biopsy performed on the breast for some other reason. *Pleomorphic* means that the LCIS cells look more atypical under the microscope than the usual case of LCIS.

Action Items

Action Items

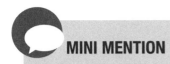

MINI MENTION

Pathology! While all tests are important, later in my journey I realized pathology is critical. There's no questioning the pathology. Pathology is fact so do your best to get a second opinion from different pathologists and make sure they are in different hospitals, not within the same practice.

While this sounds a little crazy even as I write it, I was so in disbelief that I was diagnosed with breast cancer, as I have written. After all, I looked great and felt great. I thought, *Hm. What if they mixed up my slides with someone else's?* Truly, you may go to no ends to disprove your diagnosis, which is what I did. Thus, I wanted my two biopsies reviewed. But initially, I wasn't aware: there's a pathologist? Focused on a gazillion other things with my breast and plastic surgeon (and anesthesiologist, more on that later). it wasn't until that crazy thought hit that I also thought, *Hm, pathology?*

Pathology is one of the most important factors in determining a diagnosis. It is the hard evidence which shows the presence of disease. Here there are no false positives like with the MRI. There is no gray area: it's either you have the disease or you do not, and it can show the extent of disease. It is one of the determinants of your treatment options, so you must have the most accurate report of your results.

However! Remember, as I shared with you earlier, this also might not show the entire picture as those two biopsies both missed extracting the cells that, after my mastectomy, were determined to be invasive cancer cells! As I was told by doctors, biopsies pull only a sampling of your tissues' cells.

Action Items

Action Items

When you're going for your second opinion, you will need copies of your pathology report and the actual slides with your tissue samples. While in most cases you can retrieve those from the medical records department by simply filling out a form, in some cases you may need to go directly to the pathology department located someplace else. Here you will receive your actual slides. Either way, when you make your additional appointments, leave yourself enough time to get your paper reports and slides; this may take a few days.

Sandra Lee, celebrity chef and New York Governor Andrew Cuomo's partner, just one year younger than me at forty-eight, received a diagnosis of DCIS.[7] She also did not have the BRCA gene, but her DCIS was in fact picked up by her mammogram. She ultimately chose to have a double mastectomy. Ms. Lee, like most, said she never wanted to deal with this again.

So after these two high-profile celebrity women came out and shared their stories so publicly, I began to do some research on celebrities and breast cancer. Some of you, like me, may have grown up watching *Married with Children*, and I came across an article that stated that in spring 2008, a star of that show, Christina Applegate, was diagnosed with breast cancer in her left breast at age thirty-six.[8] As a daughter of a breast cancer survivor, she was vigilant about getting mammograms. However, it was her doctor who, due to the denseness of her breasts, recommended she get an MRI, and it "lit up." He then performed a biopsy, which tested positive for breast cancer. Ms. Applegate attributes that early detection of her breast cancer to the MRI. Thus the importance of the MRI! She too had a biopsy of her

Action Items

Action Items

lymph nodes to make sure it had not spread. It was only after she received the news she had the BRCA gene (and given that her mother was a breast cancer survivor) that Ms. Applegate decided to have a double mastectomy. Like many others, she said she simply wanted to be free and clear and not have to worry again. Applegate is a passionate advocate for the MRI.

MINI MENTION

Researching insurance is often a "movement" by many that pushes things forward. I am hoping that this book will shed light on how important it is that women, regardless of diagnosis, can have access under their health insurance plans to receive at least one MRI as part of their preventative breast care.

In seeking to research what is covered and allowable, I came across densebreast-info.org.[9] While this resource is focused on those women with dense breasts, it's interesting as it has a state-by-state legislation map, noting various legislation and regulation pertaining to state insurance law and insurance coverage.

It too posts a question on its "For Patients" section of the website: "Is My Mammogram Enough?" Further, the organization shares that breast density is one of many known risk factors for breast cancer. Greater density not only increases the risk of cancer, it also makes it more difficult to detect cancer with a mammogram. There are additional screening tools available and factors to consider for each. Additional screening may lead to additional

Action Items

Action Items

testing (such as follow-up or biopsy) for findings that ultimately are not cancer. Insurance coverage may vary.

I also came across actress Angelina Jolie, who in spring 2013 chose to have a double mastectomy. She wrote an op-ed in the *New York Times* titled "My Medical Choice."[10] Here she shared her journey in hopes of helping others. I sensed that, at least in part, it also was written to address some backlash and controversy that surrounded her decisions at the time. Some thought it would start a trend of unnecessary breast surgery procedures and that she was taking too drastic of a step by getting a preventive double mastectomy. Later on, she chose her next preventative surgery, the removal of her ovaries and fallopian tubes. I say it's *never your business* to decide what is best for someone else unless you *walk in their shoes*! What made her story so unique is she chose this while having no diagnosis of breast or other cancers. But she tested positive for the BRCA gene, and this sharply increased her risk of developing both breast cancer and ovarian cancer. And given that her mother died of ovarian cancer at fifty-six, Ms. Jolie was taking no chances. She was choosing her life and her family over her breasts. This story, when it broke, addressed this debated question: How much treatment is too much, and how much is not enough? Her decision drove quite a bit of controversy in both the medical field and the public. And in fact, her story was addressed in the same *Time* magazine article[11] that I read just after I got my mastectomy.

While this may have been a difficult decision, she chose life and her family and children over her breasts. Jolie chose to have her surgery at the Pink Lotus Breast Center in Los Angeles. When I was preparing for surgery, she had publicly released

Action Items

Action Items

some of the things she did to prepare. I found this comforting and helpful and have listed the Pink Lotus Breast Center information in the resources section of this book.

MINI MENTION

Christina Applegate publicly stated that, just before her double mastectomy, she staged her "first and last nude photo shoot." Ironically, days before my surgery—I don't know if this stayed somewhere in my unconscious mind that I had read her story weeks earlier—I thought, *This will be the last I see of my right breast.*

And the first time in my life I will be losing a body part! A body part I've had for forty-nine (okay, almost fifty) years!

So at this point I too staged a photo shoot of my breasts. What's even funnier is out of all the women I spoke with from breast friends to doctors to friends, not one had mentioned this idea of taking a photo. Who did? Yes, one of my BFFs who is . . . a guy! It was so crazy. It was a few days before my surgery, and Peter and I were on the phone. Out of the blue he says, "Hey, make sure you take a picture." I quickly replied, "Been there, done that." Too funny.

PS: Now fully recovered, they look great! *And yours will too.*

When I was first diagnosed, it was truly an emotional roller coaster. One day I felt empowered and hopeful; the next I would feel exhausted and resigned. I still could not believe this was happening to me, someone who looked healthy and felt great. It was a bag of crazy, mixed emotions. It was encouraging to hear

Action Items

Action Items

from these celebrities who chose to go public with their very private and personal stories. Not knowing them personally but from television and seeing them so often, I felt a connection to them, comforted and grateful that they chose to put their stories out there and keep breast cancer in the spotlight.

They let us know that:

- Celebrity or not, this can and does happen to anyone.

- By sharing their stories so publicly, we are not alone.

- No matter how much money you have, or even with access to the "best" doctors, mistakes happen.

As one of my doctors told me, "Medicine is not 100 percent."

So it's to up to us as patients to be informed consumers to ask questions, research (based on science and facts), get multiple opinions, and be prepared. However, note this caveat: make sure not to use seeking multiple opinions as a form of delay or denial. It's a tough balance between figuring out in whose hands you will literally be putting your life and your breasts and how long you will take before actually getting treated.

Remember, when seeking out doctors, don't let anyone make you feel uncomfortable or feel guilty for asking questions or seeking out other opinions. It is *your* body and *your* health. Healthcare is a business, and your business is looking out for *you*. Then when it's time to make those difficult decisions, you will be 100 percent prepared and confident with your knowledge that you made the right choices. You will not look back with doubt as you will know you've done everything you could.

Use your instincts and listen to your gut, just as I did with my pinprick, which tipped me off that something was just not right. And with that, speaking of gut, let's talk foods, environment,

Action Items

Action Items

and the lifestyles choice we make and how they may impact our overall health and breast health. This next chapter is another who knew, in that who knew along the journey having been diagnosed with breast cancer, I'd be thinking about those things? Just a final thought on this chapter.

 MINI MENTION

Please be your own advocate and do your own science- and fact-based research; don't let any doctor tell you otherwise. I don't remember exactly how it was worded, but I actually had a doctor tell me, "Arlene, don't do your own research." I'm telling you, make sure you *do* your own research. Make sure you *do* question your doctors, and make sure they *do* answer your questions—all of them. And *do not* be intimidated; they are simply people too.

When I was telling a good friend about the second and third options I was seeking, she surprised me with a questioning tone in her voice. She said, "Arlene, it's like you're shopping around." I was like, "I sure am!" Think about the detailed questions we ask when shopping for an apartment, house, car, or even just takeout food! The doctors you choose (hopefully covered in your healthcare plan) will literally have your life in their hands. And likely you will be with that healthcare "team" for three, six, nine, or twelve months—or even for life! They will become your extended family. This is a very intimate healthcare issue. And by the way, surgery may very well be the most expensive "purchase" you make in your lifetime, so choose wisely.

Action Items

Action Items

Do not feel guilty or bad for getting other opinions; just make sure not to use seeking multiple opinions as a form of delay or denial and end up doing nothing! I got three opinions, and that's not including the myriad doctors I conferred with before making my final decisions. I even met with the anesthesiologist, and that's a story in itself. (Again, more about that later.)

MINI MENTION

At a top hospital in New York City early on in the process, I met with a potential surgeon. He was excellent. Toward the end of our appointment, I said, "I'd like to meet with a plastic surgeon here as well, should I need." He said—and this is a direct quote—"Well, unless you're doing your surgery at our hospital, I can't set that up for you." Really! Well, I ended up *not* choosing to do my surgery at that hospital and did not need to meet with their plastic surgeon. But mark my words, if I had wanted to meet with that plastic surgeon I would have. Do not be intimated. You are, in fact, a paying customer!

MINI MENTION

Just when I was resigned to removing my breast and it was now literally weeks before my scheduled

Action Items

Action Items

mastectomy, my mom called. She said she just saw a doctor on television talking about breast cancer and that this woman was the chief breast surgeon at a prominent hospital. Now, I'd been to that hospital, and that doctor's name was not on the door. By this time, I was exhausted and like, *Whatever. How many more doctors can I see?* But then that nagging feeling of hope came over me: *What if she's the one who will tell me I don't have to remove my breast, and this is not cancer?* She did not, thankfully; remember, they did not find the invasive cancer until after my surgery. But the point is, when I called this doctor's office, the receptionist answered. I said I'd like to make an appointment immediately to get another opinion. She put me on hold. *Waiting . . . waiting . . . waiting.* She then got back on the line and said, "The doctor doesn't do second opinions." "Really?" I said. I will say, by this time, with a trail of doctors behind me, I had realized—as I'd had a similar reaction from an earlier appointment at another doctor's office—that you don't tell doctors they are not your first choice. But, exhausted and desperate, it just slipped out. Needless to say I was in that office the next morning with gal pal Anita. The doctor was amazing. She spent ninety minutes with us.

The point: Do your due diligence and research, research, research! Get as many opinions as you need to feel comfortable. Never take "no" or "we can't help you" for an answer! You are the customer. Healthcare is a business, and *your* business *is taking care of you!*

Action Items

Action Items

It was at this moment, at this very last doctor's appointment, searching desperately to hear that I didn't have to cut off my right breast, that for the first time, I *cried*. The first time in this entire journey! Anita made mention of this when we walked out. Thinking back, I realized I was defeated. There were no more appointments, there were no more tests, and there were no more doctors to visit—at least in Manhattan; I had seen them all. In fact, there were no more options; this was it. I had fought the good fight. I finished the race—and DCIS had won. I knew the reality: I was headed for surgery.

"No one can make you feel
inferior without your consent."

—*Eleanor Roosevelt*[12]

Action Items

Action Items

NOTES

"There's no such thing as junk food. There's junk and there's food."

—*Mark Hyman, MD*

Chapter Five
Are We a Product of What We Eat, Our Environment, and Lifestyle Choices?

J ust as we can take ownership and control of our breast cancer diagnosis and empower ourselves, with the same focus, determination, and commitment, we can look around at the choices we make on a daily basis that may influence our health in a healthy or not-so-healthy way.

For instance, we know that smoking can cause lung cancer and is riddled with more than four thousand chemicals, of which more than seventy are known to cause, initiate, or promote cancer (called carcinogens),[1] but people *choose to smoke anyway*. We know that while the sun's rays may make us feel good and get that summer sun-kissed glow in the short term, in the long-term exposure to the sun may cause wrinkles and age spots in our later years, accelerate the aging process, and increase the risk for developing skin cancer.[2] Yet we lather on the oil and bake ourselves on the beach to obtain that perfect tan. While we know stress is not good for us as we strive to juggle priorities and climb the corporate ladder, raise children, and manage a home, we also know that stress left unchecked can contribute to many health problems such as high blood pressure, heart disease, obesity, and diabetes.[3]

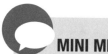

MINI MENTION

So while I don't want to digress too much, I'm compelled to share an experience I had with stress years back as it was such a huge eye opener. I believe it literally exhibited itself and affected me physically. While most of my life I've been blessed with amazing career opportunities and choices, in one position I sat at a desk from the moment I arrived in the office (sometimes 6 a.m.) to the moment I left (sometimes past 6 or 7 p.m.). I was on the computer typing away furiously, working for hours on end with no break, rarely leaving my desk to use the restroom, let alone making time for lunch. The work was completely mundane and unfulfilling, and I knew I had to go! I was miserable and had to find another opportunity *and quickly.*

It was one night while sleeping that I was awakened by an intense pain occurring in my right hand and up and down my arm. It was a pain I had never felt before and it continued on for weeks. I ignored it, thinking—hoping—it would just go away. Until it started to happen during the day as well. It became truly debilitating. I started to have trouble concentrating and focusing, but I kept pushing on. After speaking with a few friends to get their "diagnosis," the consensus was it sounded like

Action Items

Action Items

carpal tunnel syndrome. Then researching carpal tunnel symptoms, it appeared the manifestations I was having exhibited themselves exactly as that syndrome!

My breaking point to go to the doctors finally came (because I didn't have time or, frankly, I didn't make time or my health a priority) when the pain became so overwhelming both during the night and day, and with a three-day holiday weekend approaching, President's Day, I thought I simply couldn't go on. That Friday morning, I called my doctor and begged to see him; he got me in to see a specialist. The specialist confirmed it appeared to be severe symptoms of carpal tunnel. He gave me a cortisone shot which, thankfully, immediately helped relieve the pain. Now after 6 p.m. on a Friday, it was dark by this time and also happened to be snowing as I headed to the medical supply store before closing to purchase the arm brace the specialist recommended. I was desperate to do everything he said to ease the pain.

The following week he had me back for several unpleasant tests. One test shot out little electric volts, and the other prodded my arm and hand with tiny needles. He called a week later and said, "All tests came back completely negative for carpal tunnel." Yet I continued to exhibit the signs. I thought, *Hm, great news, but how can that be?* I headed back in for another cortisone shot, and he recommended I see a physical therapist and continue to wear the arm brace and come back in in a few weeks if things persisted. They did!

In the meantime, I had been actively interviewing and found a wonderful job opportunity. I gave notice at

Action Items

Action Items

my outgoing job and took a few weeks' break between jobs. It was not long after, within the short time span after I gave notice, that the pain *completely* went away. When I went back to check in with the physical therapist for one last visit, I recall him literally jumping out of his chair saying, "My god, you look so rested." I knew I was stressed out but didn't realize how much and that it had shown on my face.

The point in sharing this is that, in the same fashion as dealing with breast cancer, I persevered and took action and, thankfully, listened to my body about that pinprick. We must listen to our bodies about everything always! Not to be a hypochondriac, but to stay tuned in, we must take care of ourselves body, mind, and spirit.

Now could that timing have been coincidence? Maybe. But the bottom line, thinking back, what became truly clear is that if we don't stay tuned in to our bodies, acknowledging the signs, and assessing what's going on in and around us, unaddressed stress can *literally* make us sick. And by the way, I have never had those symptoms again!

Certainly, there are some things that affect our health that we may not have as much ability to control. Maybe it's where our parents raised us, perhaps in an urban city environment like Manhattan or Los Angeles where we were likely to encounter more smog, car fumes, and ambient air pollution versus, say, living in Vermont or Wyoming where the air is cleaner. Or our work environment may affect our health, perhaps

ACTION ITEMS

ACTION ITEMS

working in a more industrial type of construction job outdoors where there may be more safety risks.

Then there are factors completely out of our control. The clearest of cases: Tuesday, September 11, 2001. I had been working at the New York Stock Exchange for about two years. After coming out of the 2 Train exit on Wall Street, I looked down at my watch and it said 9:04 a.m. As I stepped out, I noticed there were 8 1/2 × 11 sheets of paper falling out of the sky . . . and then I encountered mayhem with people running in every direction. I heard someone say something about the Trade Center. I still have pictures from that day as I headed over some blocks and then stood there, mesmerized, at what I was looking at: the towers were literally engulfed in flames. Some gut feeling immediately told me to get out of there and head back to the Exchange, so I did.

I recall next standing with friends in front of our 20 Broad Street entrance at about 9:50 a.m., and there began a rumbling I'll never forget. It was a *thunderous* roar. We didn't know it at the time, but that noise was the Trade Center buildings beginning their collapse. We watched as that *monstrous* gray cloud of pulverized matter that so many got caught up in swooped swiftly around the buildings and came straight at us as we ran into 20 Broad. Then inside, hunkered down on the trading floor, we watched in horror the news being telecast on hundreds of flat panel television screens. These were positioned on and around each of our trading posts; the destruction was literally happening right outside our doors!

It was at 12:10 p.m. that I remember vividly Richard Grasso, our CEO, coming on the overhead mic of the exchange trading floor telling us it was okay to leave. Then, seconds later, he came

Action Items

Action Items

on to say it was okay to stay as well. I remember thinking, *No one knows what to do, even the rich and powerful.*

Having an amazing job that I absolutely loved, I stayed for four more years. Our team went back on the following Monday, just six days after the attacks. For weeks and months after I remember breathing in horrible smells and fumes; each day they'd hose down the buildings and streets with water. I remember having constant headaches but never thought too much about them. I just kept working; I loved my job.

There is no way to know what I breathed in that day as I set foot in the streets, into a deafening silence. Into a *gray snow* (literally) that was inches high and covered every street, building, and car as I walked up the East Side to 14th Street; we were not allowed to walk up the West Side. I thanked God as I was alive. I could walk. And when was it during those next four years, *that day, those weeks and months* that followed of breathing in the more than four hundred tons[4] of pulverized concrete, glass, and asbestos, as well as poisonous gases and other dangerous substances that set in motion the development of my breast cancer?

This chapter, much like this book, came about by accident. While I am not a doctor, nutritionist, or psychologist and will leave that to the many outstanding experts in those fields, I *am* writing this chapter as a person who has common sense. And I am writing this chapter as a person who, since my diagnosis of breast cancer and through my journey, has developed a heightened awareness about overall health and how we to a great extent have control over keeping ourselves in health.

I have found on this journey, when you have a sudden disruption in life, like a breast cancer diagnosis, that one

Action Items

Action Items

comes to a complete *halt*. It is then that we really begin to examine and take notice of our behaviors and what is happening in and around us. In this chapter I simply want to plant seeds that may be of immediate help to you along your journey.

As I've shared earlier on in the preface, when I was diagnosed, I started to think, *We have no breast cancer in the family. We have no cancer at all. The genetic test for the BRCA gene was negative for mutations.* It was that article in the Cancer Research UK science blog[5] that highlighted, in part, Angelina Jolie's diagnosis and her inheritance of the BRCA gene. It went on to state:

> Only a small proportion—about one in 20 (5 percent)— of the 50,000 women diagnosed with breast cancer every year carries an inherited gene fault like BRCA 1, and . . . most breast cancers arise from *genetic damage that accumulates over a person's lifetime and that's why age is the biggest risk factor.*

As I shared, this article haunted me. I thought, *Genetic damage?* How would time and age negatively affect my genes and *when*, in my forty-nine years, did they get damaged? And *who knew* genes can *change? Gosh*, I thought*, our family lives well into our late eighties and nineties. What's in store for me down the road, given the blessing of genetic longevity in our family?*

After receiving my diagnosis and making the rounds to meet with various doctors—and getting my second and third opinions—I would ask them about that science blog and note that "genetic damage accumulating over a person's lifetime and age is the biggest risk factor," and they pretty much confirmed this: it can happen with age.

ACTION ITEMS

ACTION ITEMS

But not one doctor ever spoke about the *why, when,* and, *how* that this genetic damage may occur or that we may play a factor in keeping or not keeping ourselves healthy. And with everything else going on, including myriad tests, doctors' appointments, and a busy work season, I let it go *for the moment.*

PRE-DIAGNOSIS: A NUTRITIONIST AND PRIMARY CARE PHYSICIAN (PCP) ENCOUNTER

It was pure irony that in January, two months before my diagnosis in March, as I was approaching the big five-oh with a birthday in August, that I sought out a nutritionist and was in the market for a new primary care doctor since mine had retired. Turning fifty, I started to think, *I want to make sure that I not only live long but live healthy to the very last moment on this earth!* I wanted to live my absolute best! I wanted to address the fact that I had been trying to shed that infamous five pounds (okay, ten . . . okay, fifteen-ish) forever. I wanted it off! And for months I had a chronic ache on the bottom of my feet that was becoming unbearable, particularly after sitting a long time or getting out of bed in the morning. Friends shared their "diagnosis" of the same, and it sounded like symptoms of plantar fasciitis.[6] Whatever it was, I wanted the pain gone.

So it was in my first meeting with the nutritionist in mid-January (as we had talked on the phone prior to our appointment) that she asked I come prepared with a food journal of the meals I ate, including breakfast, lunch, dinner, and snacks. We discussed my weight goals and reviewed my food choices and eating habits. She took my weight and, toward the end of our two-hour appointment, suggested a range of calories that would help set me up for successful weight loss. Last, I asked if she knew of a good primary care doctor. She

Action Items

Action Items

asked if I had any preferences and, shooting off my list to her, she said she knew a PCP focused on health and wellness, supplements, and integrative medicine (IM). While I wasn't familiar with the term *IM*, in reality I had been practicing it, in part, for some time.

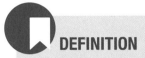

DEFINITION

INTEGRATIVE MEDICINE[7]
Healing-oriented medicine that takes account of the whole person, including all aspects of lifestyle. It emphasizes the therapeutic relationship between practitioner and patient, is informed by evidence, and makes use of all appropriate therapies.

So I was off to meet with my new PCP. I shared with him during this first visit that I was referred by the nutritionist and was looking to him for guidance on how to lose weight, identify the cause of that pain on the bottom of my feet, and how to live my *absolute best* after fifty! He asked me these questions:

1. What is your blood type?

2. How much dairy do you eat?

3. Have you ever tried a vegetarian or vegan diet?

By the end of our appointment, he suggested cutting back on dairy as well as cutting back on my sugar intake and refined and processed foods. He went on to say that I should read The *Blood Sugar Solution* by Dr. Mark Hyman[8] and check out the website PCRM.org (Physicians Committee for Responsible Medicine).[9]

ACTION ITEMS

ACTION ITEMS

THE PHYSICIANS COMMITTEE FOR RESPONSIBLE MEDICINE (PCRM.ORG)

This was the first I had heard of PCRM, and what stood out for me was its mission regarding patient empowerment and taking control of one's health. As my new PCP asked, "Did you ever try a vegetarian or vegan diet?" this website has extensive information on vegetarian and vegan diets, including a 21-day Kickstart Vegan Diet. Now I must be honest, I did try it but was not able to sustain it. I have become so accustomed to my usual Western-type diet and dieting practices that I felt completely lost in the supermarkets and planning out my meals, even with their well-outlined guide. I found it difficult, and with so much else going on, it completely overwhelmed me. So while I had given up becoming a vegetarian (for the time being), I did learn a great deal from PCRM and find it an excellent resource for health and nutrition information and guidance. I urge you to check it out.

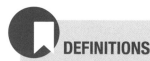

DEFINITIONS

THE PHYSICIANS COMMITTEE FOR RESPONSIBLE MEDICINE (PCRM.ORG)

The Physicians Committee is leading a revolution in medicine—putting a new focus on health and compassion. The Physicians Committee combines the clout and expertise of more than 12,000 physicians with the dedicated actions of more than 175,000 members across the United States and around the world. They are dramatically changing the way doctors treat chronic diseases,

Action Items

Action Items

such as diabetes, heart disease, obesity, and cancer. By putting prevention over pills, doctors are empowering their patients to take control of their own health. And they are also building a new way of viewing research. Since 1985, the Physicians Committee has been working for alternatives to the use of animals in medical education and research and advocating for more effective scientific methods.

REFINED FOODS[10]

These are foods altered from their original state. In exchange for altering the texture of the original grain or sugar, nutrients are lost and shelf life is generally increased.

REFINED CARBOHYDRATES[11]

These are rapidly absorbed into the bloodstream and cause risky spikes in blood sugar and insulin levels. Most common chronic diseases of Western civilization have been tied to these types of (deliciously addictive) carbohydrates; therefore, it is wise to keep them to a minimum. Refined carbohydrates are forms of sugars and starches that don't exist in nature. They do come from natural whole foods, but they have been altered in some way through processing to "refine" them. Processing methods include industrial extraction, concentration, purification, and enzymatic transformation. It's easy for most of us to identify sugars because they taste sweet and usually come in the form of crystals, syrups, or powders.

Action Items

Action Items

PROCESSED FOODS[12]

Processed foods are often high in unhealthy fats. They usually contain cheap fats and refined seed and vegetable oils (like soybean oil) that are often hydrogenated, which turns them into trans fats. Vegetable oils are extremely unhealthy, and most people are eating way too much of them already.

MINI MENTION

Who knew I'd be making a reference to the book of Daniel in the Old Testament given a breast cancer diagnosis and written in a chapter on food and lifestyle choices?

The point here is in the Old Testament book of Daniel, which some believe was written in the second century BC, there is a passage (1:1-16)[13] that gives an account of how Daniel, a Jew, is exiled to Babylon. And it's upon his arrival there he is chosen to be placed, in time and after training, into the service of the Babylonian king. Daniel was given a new name and assigned a daily amount of food and wine from the king's table. But not wanting to defile himself with the royal food and wine, which was not of Jewish diet, he asked the guard whom the chief official had appointed over himself and a few others to "[p]lease test your servants for ten days: give us nothing but vegetables to eat and water to drink. Then compare our appearance with that of the young men who eat the royal food, and treat

ACTION ITEMS

ACTION ITEMS

your servants in accordance with what you see." The official agreed and tested them in this way for the ten days. And so it was at the end of that period that they looked healthier and better nourished than the men who ate the royal food. So the guard took away their choice food and the wine they were to drink and gave them vegetables instead!

The point is even then, more than two thousand years ago, *it was pretty clear what may be best for us!*

WHAT'S YOUR BLOOD TYPE HAVE TO DO WITH IT?

During this appointment, the doctor asked me, "What is your blood type?" I immediately recalled a book that my beloved Aunt Hedy gave me that focused on exactly that. It had been given to me at least fifteen years ago. So right after this appointment I went home to search my library, and I found and dusted off *Eat Right 4 Your Type* by Dr. Peter J. D'Adamo.[14] This book outlines each blood type—O, A, B, AB—and gives a historical background and suggests highly beneficial foods for each blood type as well as what foods to avoid. This book says, right on the front cover, "Diet Solution to Staying Healthy, Living Longer, and Achieving Your Ideal Weight." Isn't it a great irony that so often we have the answers right in front of us?

I found it fascinating; this book addressed the history of blood types and genes. As my blood type is A+ (of course it is), I went on to read that "[t]ype A blood initially appeared somewhere in Asia or the Middle East between 25,000 and 15,000 BC and in response to new and different lifestyle[s], diet, and environmental conditions[,] the Type A was born and

Action Items

Action Items

eventually the gene for Type A blood spread beyond Asia and the Middle East into Western Europe."[15]

I flipped to the chapter on type A, and what immediately popped out was this: *A's thrive on vegetarian diets.* Dairy foods are poorly digested by type As, and it went on to note that type As should get their foods in as natural a state as possible: fresh, pure, and organic.

Now while my new PCP was not aware of my blood type yet, I thought how ironic it was that the exact things he shared with me not to do *for most of my life, I had been doing!* In particular, while I had some knowledge about organic foods, mostly what I knew about buying organic was that, at least in Manhattan, it is much more expensive than nonorganic foods. I always felt why pay more money? Boy, did I have a lot to learn! And dairy? I had been drinking it most of my life. What could be wrong with dairy?

DAIRY

Dairy's good for you, right? I thought back to my new PCP asking me, "How much dairy do you eat?" I proudly shared that I drank a gallon of milk a week—the healthier version, skim milk, of course. I have low-fat yogurt or cottage cheese with my fruit and eat and *love* cheese, but only low fat. My dad (and our family) is a big milk drinker, and he always said milk is healthy and full of calcium for strong bones. Right? I thought, *Why is my doc asking me about dairy?*

It was, however, after this appointment—doing everything in my type A fashion, big and bold, without even researching anything further—that I took his advice and immediately stopped drinking milk and drastically cut back on all dairy including my favorite low-fat cheeses, yogurt, and cottage cheese. I noticed

ACTION ITEMS

ACTION ITEMS

something unbelievable happen: in less than one week, after three days going cold turkey on milk and drastically limiting all dairy products that I'd eaten seemingly forever, after months and months of tightness, the pain on the bottoms of my feet *was completely gone.* I had been drinking a gallon of milk a week—at least—up to this point. Now, could it have been a fluke or coincidence? Maybe. But all I know is as I put a hard halt on dairy in my diet, I felt an immediate improvement, and this brought much needed relief.

I started to research dairy further. Here are a few *who knews?*:

- I came across an article that said American dairy farmers have been injecting cows for years with a genetically engineered bovine *growth hormone* called rBGH[16] to increase milk production. Then, due to forced milk production, the cows succumb to udder infection, and these are treated with antibiotics, which end up in our milk!

- Another article I read referenced a book, *The Cheese Trap*, by Neal Barnard, MD.[17] It addressed how dairy cows are kept pregnant most of the year, and as a result, their milk has increased estrogen levels. *Engineered growth hormones*, antibiotics, increased estrogen.

- As I continued to research dairy, the word *inflammation* kept popping up. Several articles I came across noted dairy was one of the top foods in the American diet that causes inflammation[18] and that it is highly inflammatory for many people. And more processing, like "skimming," does not make it any healthier, only more inflammatory. Milk is one of the most inflammatory foods in our diet, second to gluten.

Action Items

Action Items

Had my dad been wrong all along? As I kept reading, I found that contrary to popular belief and advertisement, bone strength does not come from consuming milk and other dairy products but from plant foods.[19]

And The China study,[20] which I learned about post–surgery from my oncologist, stated:

> In fact, dietary protein proved to be so powerful in its effect that we could turn on and turn off cancer growth simply by changing the level consumed. Furthermore, the amounts of protein being fed were those that we humans routinely consume. We didn't use extraordinary levels, as is so often the case in carcinogen studies. But that's not all. We found that not all proteins had this effect. What protein consistently and strongly promoted cancer? Casein, which makes up 87 percent of cow's milk protein, promoted all stages of the cancer process. What type of protein did not promote cancer, even at high levels of intake? The safe proteins were from plants, including wheat and soy. As this picture came into view, it began to challenge and then to shatter some of my most cherished assumptions.[21]

Needless to say, all of these *who knews* got me thinking about my choices through the years (as they may now be doing for you). Had my dad been wrong all his life, or have times just changed—from farm-fresh bottled milk delivered to your doorstep to mass-produced, genetically engineered milk laden with antibiotics ensuring maybe the best economic outcomes for companies but with complete disregard for the cow's health and the human beings drinking it? *Hm.* Just sayin'!

ACTION ITEMS

ACTION ITEMS

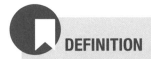

DEFINITION

THE CHINA STUDY[22]

First published in 2005, this is a book that examines the relationship between the consumption of animal products (Including dairy) and chronic illnesses such as coronary heart disease, diabetes, breast cancer, prostate cancer, and bowel cancer. The authors conclude that people who eat a wholefood, plant-based/vegan diet—avoiding all animal products, including beef, pork, poultry, fish, eggs, cheese, and milk, and reducing their intake of processed foods and refined carbohydrates—will escape, reduce, or reverse the development of numerous diseases. They write that eating foods that contain any cholesterol above 0 mg is unhealthy.

SUGAR!

While, in a general sense, I knew ingesting more sugar isn't good for, let's say, losing weight (which is why I always focused on it), I had no idea how truly *toxic* sugar is to our bodies. And how difficult it is to digest. After my new PCP suggested it, I went to the bookstore and found *Blood Sugar Solution* by Mark Hyman. Dr. Hyman's book is yet another resource that promotes self-education and empowering ourselves. He writes that we need to stop managing our symptoms and instead find a way to treat the underlying causes of illness.

So I did more research on sugar. Here are a few more of those *who knew?* facts:

- Dr. Hyman says sugar is toxic and that some animal studies show sugar is eight times more addictive than cocaine. And,

Action Items

Action Items

while the sugar industry tries to sell us on the fact that sugar is natural because it comes from sugarcane, it is simply not the case with all sugars, especially those that have undergone the refining process.

- Further, Dr. Mark Hyman, in an article called "Top 10 Big Ideas: How to Detox from Sugar,"[23] notes, "The facts are in, the science is beyond question. Sugar in all its forms is the root cause of our obesity epidemic and most of the chronic disease sucking the life out of our citizens and our economy—and, increasingly, the rest of the world. You name it, it's caused by sugar: heart disease, cancer, dementia, type 2 diabetes, depression, and even acne, infertility and impotence."

Yes, cancer. Then I started to research the words *sugar* and *cancer* together.

- On my website I posted a link to a Ted Talk I came across titled "Cancer Loves Sugar."[24] Wow, and that is scary. Again, as I have shared, ignorance *was* once bliss. While I love my candy corn during Halloween and my colorful sugarcoated marshmallow bunnies on Easter, the fact is once you are stricken with a disease and then honestly look in the mirror, there's no going back. Or if we do, we are now informed and make a choice to eat what we want, knowing it may not be healthy for us!

- I came across an article referenced in *Medical News Today*: "Sugar and Cancer: A Surprise Connection or 50-Year Coverup?"[25] This and documents by the Sugar Research Foundation suggest that knowledge of a possible link between sugar and cancer goes back as far as the 1960s.

ACTION ITEMS

ACTION ITEMS

- A report on NBC News[26] noted that researchers may be able to explain how sugar might fuel the growth of cancer. They say it boils down to one type of sugar in particular: fructose. Tests in mice show a possible mechanism for how it happens. The findings, published in the journal *Cancer Research*, support studies that suggest people who consume more sugar have a higher risk of cancer—*especially breast cancer*. "A lot of patients are told it doesn't matter what you eat after you are diagnosed with cancer. This preliminary animal research suggests that it does matter," said Lorenzo Cohen of the University of Texas MD Anderson Cancer Center, who worked on the study. The findings add one more piece of evidence to a growing body of science that shows a Western-style diet is a major risk factor for many types of cancer.[27] Other research has shown that at least two-thirds of all cases of cancer come down to lifestyle choices: tobacco use, an unhealthy diet, and a lack of exercise.

- According to the World Health Organization (WHO), our daily added-sugar consumption should be no more than 25 grams of sugar a day.[28] That is the same recommendation from the American Heart Association (AHA), which recommends only 25 grams for women.[29] Dr. Hyman notes we're consuming, on average, 152 pounds of sugar per person every year. So, a little rusty on my math, I engaged my neighbor, Bob, who is a teacher and mathematician, and we figured out together, as we converted our pounds into grams, that we are ingesting, on average, not 25 grams but *189 grams of added sugar per day*. This is more than 500 percent the daily recommended amount according to the WHO and AHA.

Action Items

Action Items

MINI MENTION

How did we get here? How did we get so unhealthy? And when did we learn these bad behaviors?

I remember heading to a doctor's appointment at about 8 a.m. As the elevator doors opened, I got on the lift and a mom was there with her child, a boy about ten years old. And, glaringly, I noticed that this boy, at 8:00 in the morning, was drinking a regular-size can of Coke and eating a bag of potato chips! And I thought to myself, *Here is where poor eating habits begin.*

If you have never noticed—and I get it—that ignorance is bliss, check out that favorite can of soda, *any* regular soda. Yes! Just one twelve-ounce can of regular soda has about 39 grams of sugar—*in one can.* The WHO and AHA recommended daily allowance for sugar for women is 25 grams for the entire day! Can you imagine this child has already started his day over the daily recommended allowance of sugar? This gives perspective, and it's not hard to imagine when Dr. Hyman shares that we're consuming 152 pounds of sugar! Per person! Every year!

And far worse: it is this eating pattern that may very well shape a child's health, or lack of, for the rest of his or her life. I'm learning along my journey that the effects of our poor diets, our environment, exposures to various elements, our genetics, and chance and luck can create great damage. And the harm we cause in our earlier years doesn't necessarily show up until later in life as we age! But in your twenties, who thinks about their forties, fifties, or sixties?

Action Items

Action Items

Listen! I'm not saying that sometimes I don't love or crave a regular soda. But doing so now comes with the knowledge that there is a price to pay. Ignorance *was* bliss.

And we haven't even talked about the toxic food colorings and other chemicals that go into that twelve-ounce can. Go ahead: *research those ingredients!*

A TOXIC BREW

I gather that if I didn't already, I now have your attention! Or better yet, while reading this you have started to think about *your* diet or *your* current lifestyle choices. Bravo! And don't worry. We can change! And that's the good news. But as I've said, ignorance truly *was* bliss.

So as I continued to peruse websites and read about dairy and sugar, I was then led to articles about our meats, vegetables, and fruits. The more I researched, the more scary stuff I found. While never a big red meat eater—mostly chicken and fish—I found endless articles about the hormones in our meats, the pesticides sprayed on our fruits and vegetables, and the list goes on. Watch *Food, Inc.*[30]: truly frightening. Beware! You may never want to eat chicken again after seeing the treatment and processing of baby chicks. As an animal lover, honestly, it's a visual I wish I had never seen. I can't forget it; it is repulsive and inhuman. Terrible.

For a big eyeopener, check out the EWG Environmental Working Groups website. The EWG is an American environmental organization that specializes in research and advocacy in the areas of toxic chemicals, agricultural subsidies, public lands,

Action Items

Action Items

and corporate accountability.[31] I was shocked to uncover that those fabulous sales on strawberries I get so excited about at my local market come with a price! Yes, a toxic price: strawberries that are not organic are one of our fruits that contain the highest levels of pesticides.

I began to think, has the food industry been slowly poisoning us for decades? To preserve food longer and increase sales so the bottom line is better? Why do we as consumers have to pay (often) higher prices for foods that are deemed "organic" and be charged more for milk without antibiotics, for hormone-free meats, or for our fruits and vegetables not to be riddled with pesticides?

The Food and Drug Administration (FDA) is entrusted to protect our foods. As posted on the FDA website, it is noted that they are "responsible for protecting the public health by ensuring the safety, efficacy, and security of human and veterinary drugs, biological products, and medical devices; *and by ensuring the safety of our nation's food supply*, cosmetics, and products that emit radiation."[32] *Hm.* During my research, words that continually kept creeping up (in almost all the literature) were *inflammation, casein, allergies, antibiotics, hormones, pesticides, genetically engineered*—and the toxic list went on.

Reading these articles and researching all of this was quite the wakeup call for me. The more I read, the more I realized many of the foods I deemed "healthy," "low fat," and "fresh" were actually packed with sugar and carbohydrates and riddled with pesticides, hormones, and antibiotics. The dots were connecting, and those "dots" represented the fact that we *do* play a hand in keeping ourselves healthy.

I started to wonder, *Are we as consumers literally poisoning ourselves with dairy, sugar, and other poor food choices? Are our*

ACTION ITEMS

ACTION ITEMS

supermarkets, with their endless aisles of food choices, literally making us sick? It was at this moment I realized *we are in fact what we eat,* and I think we can literally eat ourselves into illness.

I challenge you, right now as you are reading this: STOP. Go to your kitchen pantry or refrigerator and take out a box of your favorite cereal, cake, soup, or container of juice or soda can. Then, yes, take a look at the (likely) long list of ingredients:

- How many ingredients are listed?

- How many ingredients can you not pronounce?

- Do you know what they *are*?

- No? *Okay, then research them!*

Yes, *now*. Go quickly, right now, on the internet. I'll wait.

You'll no doubt have likely identified preservatives, food colorings, and myriad chemicals. And sold in our favorite retail supermarkets!

What's a bit startling as well (or perhaps more disappointing) is that, along my breast cancer journey, it was only my PCP doctor (earlier on) and oncologist (whom I met with post-surgery)—and *not the nutritionist* or any other doctors—who stopped to discuss genetics, food, lifestyle, or the impact the environment may have on overall health and our genes as we age. I run a medical education conference for our cardiology team called Prevention to Intervention. While my programs focus on heart health, the word *prevention* is finally a word that is seeping into all areas of healthcare from starting at your PCP and forward and finally getting the traction and attention it deserves. In offering all my continuing medical education programs, I am proactive in working alongside our

Action Items

Action Items

physician course directors to ensure there's a session supportive of prevention and health and wellness addressing body *and* mind.

THE ONCOLOGIST: POST-SURGERY

It wasn't until meeting with the oncologist for the first time, about three weeks after surgery in July, that he reviewed my reports to confirm that they found 3.5 mm of invasive cancer and now staged my breast cancer as Stage 1A. *What a blessing,* I thought, *that I never found that "one" doctor I was looking for, begging to find, who would tell me, "Okay, Arlene, you do not need to have surgery."*

Thinking back to that article on genetic damage from the science blog I read in March, I asked him questions about genetics and cells changing and the age factor. He said to check out *The China Study*[33] by T. Colin Campbell and "The Dirty Dozen." Ouch! That was a harsh wakeup call! It's in this study they link specific diseases to diet.

In still more research, I stumbled upon the Centers for Disease Control and Prevention website and data that showed the top ten leading causes of death in the United States, with heart disease and cancer topping the chart.[34] Again I wondered: a pattern, and those "dots," continued to connect as I recognized this same list of diseases not only from *The China Study* but also from Dr. Hyman's book and myriad other resources I came across.

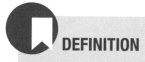

DEFINITION

THE CENTERS FOR DISEASE CONTROL AND PREVENTION[35]

CDC works 24/7 to protect America from health, safety, and security threats, both foreign and in the United

ACTION ITEMS

ACTION ITEMS

States. Whether diseases start at home or abroad, are chronic or acute, curable or preventable, human error or deliberate attack, CDC fights disease and supports communities and citizens to do the same. As the nation's health protection agency, CDC saves lives and protects people from health threats. CDC conducts critical science and provides health information that protects our nation against expensive and dangerous health threats and responds when these arise.

CAN WE HEAL OURSELVES?

As I kept researching diet and health, I recalled an article I had printed and saved in my library. I found it and, again, like with other resources, I dusted it off. I found this article on a television special one day on WNET, a public television station in New York. The special was hosted by Dr. Lissa Rankin, a physician, author, speaker, teacher, and founder of the Whole Health Medicine Institute. Dr. Rankin shared her story of how, one day, she realized she was stressed out and overworked and needed a change to heal herself—mind, body, and soul. Along with many changes she felt she needed to make, reducing stress and making a change in her diet was at the top of her list.

In the special, she referred to the Spontaneous Remission Project, a study of more than 3,500 verifiable documented cases in medical literature in which patients have been cured from seemingly "incurable" diseases either without medical treatment or without treatment deemed adequate for cure. Many of these patients were cured from terminal Stage 4 type cancers

ACTION ITEMS

ACTION ITEMS

that simply disappeared. Dr. Rankin shares that she wondered whether these could be flukes or these patients did something proactive to cure themselves.

Dr. Kelly Turner, a PhD who trained at Harvard and UC Berkeley, had that same question and wrote *Radical Remission: Surviving Cancer Against All Odds.*[36] Dr. Rankin tracked down Dr. Turner to interview her for her book *Mind Over Medicine: Scientific Proof That You Can Heal Yourself.*[37] Dr. Turner shared that she traveled the world, studying people who experienced what she calls "unexpected remissions" from Stage 4 cancer. Turner prefers the term *unexpected remissions* to *spontaneous remissions* because the word *spontaneous* implies something just happened or was luck and the patient wasn't involved in the cure. And what Dr. Turner found is these unexpected remissions *were not accidents*. In fact, she identified a common thread connecting all of these patients' stories, and there were six proactive health behaviors to which they credited their unexpected remissions. And wow—the list blew my mind. Here's the list, and guess what number one was:

1. Change your diet.

2. Deepen your spirituality.

3. Feel love, joy, and happiness.

4. Release repressed emotions.

5. Take herbs or vitamins.

6. Use intuition to help make treatment decisions.

As Turner discussed a person changing their diet, she referenced Kris Carr's *Crazy Sexy Diet*. I then researched Carr. After

Action Items

Action Items

being diagnosed with an "incurable" Stage 4 cancer, Carr fought her cancer with a vegan, largely raw, chemical-free, anti-inflammatory diet. In her book, she shares that this change of diet helped her "ignite a personal revolution and taught . . . how to participate in [my] wellbeing in the deepest level imaginable."[38] Having spent more than a decade adhering to a prevention-focused diet and lifestyle, she is doing better today than the day she was diagnosed.

While reading this, I recalled yet another book on this same type of subject matter: healing oneself. Once again, I went back to my library and really had to dust this one off: *Love, Medicine & Miracles*, by Dr. Bernie S. Siegel, written in 1986.[39] Ironically, I recall finding this book in one of my high school classes, and it caught my eye as it sat there looking lonely on a desk. I remember thinking it odd that it sat there like that. Apparently it had no owner, and after flipping through some pages and finding it quite interesting, I took it. Now more than thirty years later, as I flipped through it, I again became caught up in it. Dr. Siegel showcases his exceptional patients and how they overcame cancer through being proactive in their own care.

COMING FULL CIRCLE

While I like to open and close each chapter with a quote that somewhere along the road of life made an impression on me—as well as being pertinent to that chapter—I have to inject here a favorite quote of mine. It is actually the first quote in my quote book that I started back in 1999. It is by T.S. Eliot and reflects some very strong feelings that I hold:

> We must not cease from exploration. And at the end of all of our exploring will be to arrive where we began and to know the place for the first time.[40]

ACTION ITEMS

ACTION ITEMS

With great irony and timing, as I was rewriting this chapter, I was watching CNN's Fareed Zakaria on Sunday, November 27, 2016. Zakaria had on his show an author, Siddhartha Mukherjee, a Pulitzer Prize winner whose new book was *The Gene: An Intimate History*. It is a story of the quest to decipher the master code of instructions that makes and defines humans. At one point in the interview Mukherjee commented on breast cancer and said (I paraphrase his statement): While we are not yet there, researchers are at the forefront of identifying the exact mutations for specific diseases like breast cancer, so that they can then single out and address with direct therapy and or prevent.[41]

I was so grateful to have stumbled upon this show segment and Mukherjee's book. In great part it further validated the fact that I had made the right decision to remove my breast based on the information I researched and gathered *at that moment in time*. While DCIS is surrounded by some controversy, the bottom line is the science at this time simply cannot address the *when* or *if* of whether those bad mutated DCIS cells *will or will not* turn into invasive cancer. As all my pre-surgery biopsy tests showed only the DCIS, it was not until after my surgery and meeting with the oncologist weeks later that I found, in fact, the DCIS had turned into *invasive, "real"* cancer and then was staged as Stage 1A.

Further, after seeing this segment, I purchased Mukherjee's book. Chapter 10 of Mukherjee's book was quite relevant and addressed in part the answers to the questions I was asking. Here's an excerpt from that chapter that "clicked" for me, helping me answer those haunting questions.

Neither the genotype or the environment is the sole predictor of outcome[;] it is the intersection of genes, environment and chance. In humans a mutant BRCA

ACTION ITEMS

ACTION ITEMS

138

1 gene increases the risk for breast cancer[,] but not all women carrying the BRCA 1 mutation develop cancer. Such trigger dependent or chance dependent genes are described as having partial or incomplete penetrance i.e. even if [the] gene is inherited its capacity to penetrate into an actual attribute is not absolute. Or a gene may have variable expressivity i.e. even if the gene is inherited its capacity to become expressed as an actual attribute varies from one individual to another. One woman with the BRCA 1 mutation might develop an aggressive metastatic variant of breast cancer at age 30, another women with the same mutation might develop an indolent variant, and yet another might not develop breast cancer at all. We still do not know what causes the difference of outcomes between these three women but it is some combination of age, exposures, other genes, and bad luck. You cannot use just the genotype BRCA 1 mutation to predict the final outcome with certainty. So the final modification might read as genotype plus environment plus triggers plus chance equal phenotype. Succinct yet magisterial, this formula captured the essence of the interactions between heredity, chance, environment, variation, and evolution in determining the form and fate of an organism.[42]

9/11 CERTIFIED

Lastly, a colleague of mine in the area of public health, Francine, and I were talking about past jobs, and I shared I had worked at the New York Stock Exchange. She suggested I apply to the 9/11 WTC Health Program. Francine has experience working with the Northwell Health Queens WTC Health Program clinic,

ACTION ITEMS

ACTION ITEMS

which is part of her department and affiliated with the 9/11 WTC Health Program. I had never heard of this program. She went on to say it monitors and treats those who were in lower Manhattan on and in the days following September 11, 2001, and it does so for life. It's a program that was made into law by the James Zadroga 9/11 Health and Compensation Act of 2010 and is administered by the National Institute for Occupational Safety and Health, Centers for Disease Control and Prevention, and the U.S. Department of Health and Human Services. A wonderful and well-needed program.

In closing, it is now clear to me that we *can* impact our health either in positive or not-so-positive ways and, with *age*, we need to always take care of ourselves—body, mind, and spirit. While I started writing this book as I approached fifty in 2015, I will be fifty-five when this book releases! And I plan to be around a long while, for sure, making better choices. May we *all* choose wisely!

"We know that food is information, not just calories, and that it can upgrade your biologic software. The majority of chronic disease is primarily a food borne illness. We ate ourselves into this problem, and we have to eat ourselves out of it."

—*Mark Hyman, MD*[43]

ACTION ITEMS

ACTION ITEMS

NOTES

"What lies behind us and what lies before us are tiny matters compared to what lies within us."

—*Ralph Waldo Emerson*

Part Three
Surgery, Healing, and Let's Talk about DCIS

"Human beings are made of body, mind, and spirit. Of these, spirit is primary, for it connects us to the source of everything, the eternal field of consciousness."

—*Deepak Chopra*[1]

Chapter Six
Preparing for Surgery: Body, Mind, Spirit, Signs, and Saints

Weeks before my surgery, I had a tremendous amount of anxiety. I was absolutely terrified of going into surgery and not waking up. In thinking about the origin of this anxiety, I gathered that, aside from my appendix being removed laparoscopically more than fifteen years earlier, this was the first "official" big surgery in my life. And while I wouldn't say it out loud and tried to not even think about it, a body part—my right breast of forty-nine years (okay, almost fifty)—was going to be removed and replaced by something plastic with silicone in it. *Really!*

Now late April, I scheduled another visit to my PCP. But this visit wasn't to follow up on how my weight loss was coming or for more tips on living well, but to share with him that I'd been diagnosed with breast cancer.

Up to this point in my life, while I can think of only a time or two I could have used some medicinal help, I've never taken any type of anxiety medication. But distraught with my impending surgery, I was now seriously seeking something to relieve my growing anxiety. And if I was completely honest with myself, I was still looking, searching, hoping for that *one doctor* who would tell me, "You don't need to have your breast removed. And so it went. I walked out of his office after that appointment that day with a prescription for an anti-anxiety medication—and the name of an IM oncologist here in New York.

With my PCP telling me it was this type of doctor who takes a unique approach to medicine, he inadvertently infused in me new hope that this doctor might be that one doctor who would have a different diagnosis or treatment option for me. But it just wasn't meant to be. While I am usually 99.9 percent effective at getting in doors—as when needed my pushy type A kicks in to help—this integrative medicine specialist was booked out for three months. Despite every way that I tried to schedule an appointment to see him, it simply was not going to happen. Thank goodness; remember that, unknown at this time to my doctors and me, the DCIS *had already turned to invasive Stage 1A cancer,* and while the two mammograms and ultrasound missed the DCIS, the two needle biopsies missed the invasive cancer as well. Yep!

By this time, with a trail of doctors left behind me in the dust, and having had extensive tests and enough research to write this book (!), and through the guidance of many breast friends, all conclusions were pointing that, at this given time, given my diagnosis and current medical treatment options available, surgery was imminent and the best plan. And frankly, I didn't want to delay the surgery longer as I wanted this disease out of my body before it spread or, even worse, caused more changes as invasive cancer.

ACTION ITEMS

ACTION ITEMS

It is always interesting to me how things work out. I truly believe everything happens for a reason. And while I couldn't get an appointment to see the integrative doctor who may have said those magic words I thought I was looking for, it's often been my experience that that first step isn't necessarily the step you're meant to take. Still, it must be taken, as it leads you to that next step which may lead you to that *next* step, *which is the actual step we are meant to get to!* Got it! So, not being able to schedule an appointment with this specialist, I started researching: what exactly is integrative medicine?

It was at this moment that I recalled that the consumer-facing part of the women's heart health conference I managed—when I met Dr. Pollycove—focused on preventive and integrative medicine. So I pulled out the conference brochure and found it did indeed highlight yoga practice, bodywork, transcendental meditation, healthy eating, proper diet, exercise, and wellness. I was realizing that while I didn't know it by that term or name, I had been well familiar with and actually engaging in IM and its practices all along, as you too may now recognize.

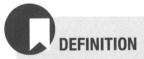

DEFINITION

INTEGRATIVE MEDICINE (IM)[2]

IM takes into account the whole person, including all aspects of lifestyle. It emphasizes the therapeutic relationship between doctor and patient, is informed by evidence, and makes use of all appropriate therapies. Both doctors and patients alike are bonding with the philosophy of integrative medicine and its whole-person approach, designed to treat the person, not just the disease. The goal

Action Items

Action Items

is to treat mind, body, and spirit, all at the same time. While some of the therapies used may be nonconventional, a guiding principle within integrative medicine is to use therapies that have some high-quality evidence to support them.

As I was researching IM, I came across the Johns Hopkins website, which was outstanding. It was here I found information on complementary and alternative medicine (CAM). Many different areas make up the practice of CAM, and many parts of one field may overlap with parts of another field. While there is extensive information one can find on this site, here's an excerpt[3]:

Traditional alternative medicine includes the more mainstream and accepted forms of therapy such as acupuncture, homeopathy, and Oriental practices. These therapies have been practiced for centuries worldwide. Traditional alternative medicine may include:

- Acupuncture

- Ayurveda

- Homeopathy

- Naturopathy

- Chinese or Oriental medicine

As I continued to research these alternative forms of medicine, I came across a most interesting article on WebMD which resonated with me, and you'll quickly see why!

ACTION ITEMS

ACTION ITEMS

In part the article highlighted a woman who had breast cancer and a myriad of other health issues. In addition to her annual checkups and testing, she made a beeline for the Duke Center for Integrative Medicine. There she learned about nutrition, fitness, yoga, tai chi, meditation, and other practices. After her diagnosis, these practices helped with her healing process and living a better quality of life. She went on to say, "I'm a type A personality, and I knew I had to do something about my lifestyle. I had to bring myself down to a type B." It was that sentence that really caught my attention and resonated so close to home for me and, while I *instinctively* knew what she meant (as a proud type A-er), I had never thought about it in that way. Being competitive and aggressive may not always be a good thing when it comes to your health. So after reading this article I looked up the definition of a type A personality.

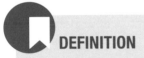

DEFINITION

TYPE A AND TYPE B PERSONALITY THEORY[4]

Type A and type B personality theory describes two contrasting personality types. In theory, personalities that are more competitive, outgoing, ambitious, impatient, and/or aggressive are labeled type A, while more relaxed personalities are labeled type B.

While I joke about being a type A personality, I started to think, *I certainly exude these qualities.* Then I started to think, *Hm, what determines how one becomes a type A?* Please, don't worry! We are not going to digress into my childhood here; this book would not end! But it is true that, later in life, I do acknowledge

ACTION ITEMS

ACTION ITEMS

that I am competitive and ambitious. I do thrive on accomplishing the goals and objectives I set for myself or those I am given. I do everything I decide to do with great energy, enthusiasm, heart, and passion, and I literally pour myself out 110 percent. I thought, *What could be wrong with that?*

SOMETIMES WE ALL NEED A WAKEUP CALL

I started to realize that when you're used to running yourself at full throttle, ninety miles per hour nonstop to obtain that elusive perfection and success in your career and all areas of life, and you're juggling work obligations, family commitments, time for significant others, friends, furry friends—just essentially busy living life on high speed—when you get ill and receive a diagnosis such as breast cancer, that diagnosis becomes a *huge* wakeup call. It makes you step back and examine life and how you're living it—*or not.*

The bottom line is I started to realize that at some point you cannot keep running at that fast of a pace without something breaking down. Even though I consider it, perhaps, "good" stress, regardless—just like a car needs refueling or an oil change—we too need tune-ups. This diagnosis was *devastating*, and it literally *slammed the brakes on my life.* And this tune-up, for me, was overwhelming as it turned out to be a full part *replacement* . . . and that part was literally the removal and replacement of my breast. If you've faced a similar diagnosis, you may be feeling the same way.

So talking about that "next step leading to that next step," it was late one night (around 3 a.m.), and I was up on the internet continuing to research IM and gaining an understanding of what it was when it popped into my mind to search for these two words together: *meditation* and *surgery.* It was then, in the

ACTION ITEMS

ACTION ITEMS

middle of the night, that I came across a blog that had a link to an audio interview and a book associated with it. The book, by Peggy Huddleston, was called *Prepare for Surgery, Heal Faster: A Guide of Mind-Body Techniques*.[5] In her book, Huddleston discusses and shares research on the positive impacts of meeting with the anesthesiologist, creating healing statements, the power of prayer, and much more.

I can't say how *hugely* helpful this book was for me in so many ways. And it came to me in perfect timing, as things always do, right? Keep alert and watch for serendipity in your life; it's likely all around you! So after listening to that audio interview Ms. Huddleston had posted on the internet, I was impressed, and I ordered the book the very next day. Within less than a week I was reading as quickly as I could. The book, in a word, is extraordinary.

DISCOVERING OUR INNER POWER

This book helped me manage my anxiety prior to surgery with meditative and relaxing techniques, and it came with two incredible relaxation CDs, but just as importantly, like *my role* in taking control of my diagnosis, like *my role* in realizing I control my lifestyle choices, this book helped me further think about *my role* in taking control of *my* preparation for surgery and *my role* in the healing process. That book was yet another catalyst to help me write this book for *you* to share helpful tips that may help you prepare for your surgery and heal your body, mind, and spirit. Here I'll share a bit of how I benefitted from her book, but this is just a very small sampling, and I truly urge you to go out and get a copy. It was truly pivotal for me and may, too, be for you.

And by the way, I never needed to fill that prescription for that antianxiety medication. I don't want to sound averse to

Action Items

Action Items

taking prescription drugs if there is a diagnosis of a condition and someone can benefit. I'm not a "delegator"; I don't want to delegate my feeling and emotions and be dependent on a drug to keep me well *if I can help myself*—especially with so many addiction concerns so prevalent in our society.

I thought, *Don't we more often than not have the power to help ourselves?* But we may not realize it, or we give up that power for an easier road or depend on others for *our* answers! I chuckle as I think about a favorite movie of mine, *The Wizard of Oz,*[6] when Dorothy is upset as the hot air balloon has left without her (near the story's end), and she now wonders how, after this entire journey following that long yellow brick road, and helping so many along the way … who will help *her* get home to Kansas? Then Glinda appears and says, "My dear, you don't need to be helped. You have always had the power all along to get home but had to find it out for yourself."[7] Like Dorothy, we too own our power; we just have to find it and believe in ourselves. And often it's in the most difficult of circumstances that we flourish and rise to the occasion and even end up surprising ourselves!

While I like to start and end each chapter with an inspired quote, here are a couple so fitting I'd like to place them here.

A woman is like a tea bag. You can't tell how strong she is until you put her in hot water.[8] —Eleanor Roosevelt

Everyone is a house with four rooms: a physical, a mental, an emotional, and a spiritual. Most of us tend to live in one room most of the time, but unless we go into every room every day, even if only to keep it aired, we are not a complete person.[9] —Indian proverb

Action Items

Action Items

MEETING YOUR HEALTHCARE TEAM CAN REDUCE ANXIETY, EVEN YOUR ANESTHESIOLOGIST

Anesthesiologist? By this time, after meeting with teams of doctors in various practices, I had not yet come across the anesthesiologist. I thought, *How could I have missed hearing about this particular doctor?* Well, to answer my question and cut myself a break, because I'd never had surgery before and was overwhelmed managing a thousand other things! I began thinking, *What exactly do they do during surgery?* And why meet with them? Let's start here!

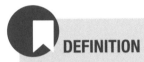

DEFINITION

ANESTHESIOLOGIST[10]

A doctor, MD or DO, who practices anesthesia. Anesthesiologists are physicians specializing in perioperative care, development of an anesthetic plan, and the administration of anesthetics. Anesthesiology is the practice of medicine dedicated to the relief of pain and total care of the surgical patient before, during, and after surgery. During the surgery, the anesthesiologist will monitor the patient's blood pressure, heart rhythm, temperature, level of consciousness, and amount of oxygen in the blood. For a general anesthetic, the anesthesiologist will monitor each breath. They may also measure the amount of blood the heart is pumping and blood pressure inside the lung vessels.

Yikes! While I thought I had done my diligence in vetting all doctors that were going to be present during my surgery, and making sure I had the best possible team, it is this doctor,

ACTION ITEMS

ACTION ITEMS

the anesthesiologist, who by definition *literally* has one's life and breath in their hands. This one person was responsible for keeping me alive! They are in charge of my vitals, my airway management (breathing), intraoperative life support, provision of pain control, and more.

Noted in Huddleston's book, a research study at Harvard Medical School showed that arranging a meeting well before surgery significantly reduced patients' preoperative anxiety.[11] Hearing about the anesthesiologist now, for the first time, and the importance of their critical role during my surgery, I was now on a new mission to—you guessed it—meet with my anesthesiologist.

Now I wanted to ensure I had the best anesthesiologist. I wanted to make sure my surgeons knew of, had worked with, and approved of my anesthesiologist. So during my next appointment I asked my plastic surgeon how I would go about meeting with the anesthesiologist; it was a simple question, I thought. He shared, "You meet with your anesthesiologist the day of your surgery." My immediate reaction: *"The day of?!"* This doctor, who plays a critical role during surgery—yes, that of keeping you alive—why wouldn't I be able to meet with them prior to the date of surgery? Asking this question to the surgeon, he gave me this analogy: it's like pilots with planes. Procedures and surgeries are everchanging, and therefore so do their schedules. Okay, I got it. I understand. Thank you very much. And that is *so* absolutely of no comfort to me, the type-A control freak riddled with anxiety who is in terror of this surgery! Still, I persisted in telling my doctor how important it was for me to meet with my anesthesiologist before the surgery.

It became clear to my plastic surgeon that I was not giving up my quest to meet the doctor in charge of keeping me

Action Items

Action Items

alive during surgery—whether my surgeon picked up on my impending fear and anxiety or he just wanted me to stop calling his office, *I really didn't care.* So after numerous follow-up calls, *voila!* I received a call for an appointment to meet with the anesthesiologist. Ask and you shall receive.

Please hold on to this for a moment; we'll come back to it.

WE NEED MORE THAN JUST CLINICAL EXPERTISE

Huddleston's book also addressed the research behind and power of healing statements read during your surgery. I was like, *What are healing statements?* They are as described are positive statements your healthcare team, usually your anesthesiologist, can read to you while you are going under, during, and coming out of anesthesia. As noted in Huddleston's book, "Research from around the world shows that—contrary to what has been commonly believed—when you are anesthetized and unconscious, you hear what is said during surgery. Furthermore, you are powerfully influenced by what you hear, much like a person under hypnosis."[12]

MINI MENTION

I went for a gynecological procedure recently to remove a polyp in my cervix, and I mentioned to the anesthesiologist that I usually have healing statements read. But this being, literally, a less-than-60-minute procedure, I didn't prepare any.

Funny enough, she said, to paraphrase, "Some crazy lady came in with that a few weeks ago." *Hm, crazy?* She was nice and chuckled in a funny way but clearly

Action Items

Action Items

didn't get it, so I'll forgive her, but I won't forget. Now not sure where that *other* "crazy lady" may have heard about healing statements, but I'm so glad other patients are taking charge, hearing about this, and doing what's best for them.

Huddleston's book goes on to cite studies and the positive impact of healing statements, from top medical centers of excellence from Emory University School of Medicine in Atlanta, Harvard Medical School in Boston to St. Thomas's Hospital in London. All show varying benefits for patients who had positive statements spoken to them, like needing less anesthesia during surgery, recovering more quickly with less pain, using less pain medications post-surgery, and, in some cases, healing more quickly.[13]

Thus, after reading this, there was no question that, in addition to meeting with my anesthesiologist to ensure they were the best doctor and would work seamlessly with the other members of my healthcare team, now I needed to make sure they were on board with and understood the importance of reading my healing statements while putting me under anesthesia, during the surgery, and while coming out of my surgery.

Let's go back to meeting with the anesthesiologist. The weeks had passed pretty quickly. While I sat in the doctor's office waiting patiently, the doctor walked in and introduced himself as the chief of anesthesiology. I was impressed that the chief of the department would take the time to meet with me, but I thought, *Is he going to be my anesthesiologist?* No, he was not. When booking the initial appointment, I was quite clear that I wanted to meet with the doctor who would be in my surgery

ACTION ITEMS

ACTION ITEMS

and talk about my healing statements. Yet upon sitting down, he began to *ask me* a lot of questions:

- What's your age?

- Have you had any surgeries before this?

- Have you ever had anesthesia?

- Have you had any reactions to anesthesia?

He was extremely nice and spent a good thirty minutes with me, but pretty much that entire time was spent on me answering *his* questions. This was not the conversation I expected and, feeling like our time was coming to an end, I was aware that he had never once addressed my healing statements. Honestly, I felt somewhat intimidated and embarrassed, like I was asking for something so unusual, and *apparently I was*, so I meekly took out my pink paper with my prepared healing statements that I'd want read to me during surgery, all nicely typed up to share with him.

It was clear I had lost him! But then I quickly realized that I never had him. There was an odd, long silence while he took on a glazed, empty, dismissive look in his eye as he took my healing statements into his hand and muttered something—which I honestly can't remember. He made me feel so uncomfortable that I think I tuned out, and then he got up and sent me on my way, never addressing what I was there to see him about in the first place: my healing statements. It was obvious to me at that point that, yes, thankfully, he and his team were going to do their very best to make sure I stayed medically alive during the surgery, to not die on their watch, but he had no interest in helping calm my anxiety. When I left his office, I felt like he thought—and frankly, he made me feel—that this was a crazy request.

Action Items

Action Items

CHAPTER SIX

A few questions went through my mind afterward as I started to second guess myself: *am I* crazy? Was I crazy in asking to meet with the anesthesiologist—the doctor in charge of keeping me alive for this very serious surgery? Was I crazy to have my healing statements read in an attempt to help ease my anxiety and possibly help me recover more quickly? The answer to my questions was the same for all of them: *no.*

Looking back, this had been the undertone, at least in part, the feeling, I got and felt from most of the doctors I met with: there was a great divide between the doctor's objectives and mine as the patient. I felt he was concerned about one thing, and that was not letting me die on his watch—and I am certainly thankful for that! But I felt he had no great concern about my overall wellness or how I felt or my expectations as a patient. There was no tremendous comfort provided, no reassurance that my healing statements would be read.

 MINI MENTION

I do understand a doctor's time and resources are limited and stretched. The irony for me is that as a healthcare educator in continuing medical education (CME) focused on helping our clinicians close the gaps between current and best practices, courses should ultimately lead to improvement of patient care and outcomes. But now, as I'm a patient, it feels like the patient has been forgotten. *I feel forgotten.*

Never giving up, after this meeting with the chief anesthesiologist I called my surgeon's office yet again to request to meet with the actual anesthesiologist who would be with me during my four-to five-hour surgery! *Voila!* One

ACTION ITEMS

ACTION ITEMS

week before my surgery I heard from Dr. Yuh, my assigned anesthesiologist. She was, in a word, awesome! While we spent maybe ten minutes on the phone, she introduced herself and *listened*. She understood the importance—to me—of having my healing statements read. I felt true sincerity, thoughtfulness, and concern for my feelings and needs. Before we ended our call, she said she would be happy to read the statements, and I would meet her on the day of surgery. For all this, I was so extremely grateful.

Fast forward to the day of surgery. As I sat in my blue gown finishing up my paperwork, Dr. Yuh walked in, and we finally met in person. I gave her my healing statements. And to be absolutely sure she was okay in reading them, I asked her, then and there, to please read one sentence: "Following this operation, you will feel comfortable, and you will heal very well."

Now feeling completely confident—at least as much as I could possibly be—I was escorted into surgery. I am so thankful for Dr. Yuh and her *outstanding care*.

TOGETHER WE ARE STRONGER

Huddleston's book also references the power of prayer and organizing a prayer group, noting a study where a computer randomly assigned patients to one group that was prayed for and another that was not and showing some remarkable outcomes for the group that was prayed for.[14]

Now I'm sure you know what I did next to further prepare myself for surgery, right? You got it: I typed up a sheet noting specifics on *what time my surgery was, when to pray for me*, and *what to pray for*, which would tie into my healing statements. I created

ACTION ITEMS

ACTION ITEMS

a list of family, friends, breast friends, colleagues, and those from my church I wanted to reach out to and asked them to pray for me. I did so by email, phone, and in person, handing out my prayer sheets. I then began to pray for myself, and my wonderful mom gave me a beautiful prayer and novena to the Infant of Prague,[15] which I prayed daily leading up to my surgery. I also prayed for my doctors and those on my surgical team (even those whose names I didn't know—I couldn't know everyone!).

WHEN TWO OR MORE GATHER YOU CAN FIND INNER POWER

When I first moved into Manhattan's Upper West Side, I joined Holy Name of Jesus Church (HNOJ) located on 96th and Amsterdam Avenue. It is a Catholic parish run by the Franciscans religious order within the Catholic Church and was founded in 1209 by Saint Francis of Assisi. I joined as I wanted to become involved and help those in the community in which I lived. After a few years teaching religious education on Sunday mornings and looking for other ways I could help, I came across an opportunity in the church bulletin asking for volunteers to serve Mass as a Eucharistic Minister, and since 2004 I have been a Eucharistic Minister.

Weeks before my surgery, as I was sharing with my church group that I would not be able to serve for some time, Gerald, one of our members, said he would coordinate a prayer service for me after Mass the following week. So that Saturday, two weeks before my surgery, after the 5:30 p.m. Mass, Father Larry and Father Matthew gathered us up, all ten of us, and led a beautiful prayer service. He had a trifold, green-colored card he gave each of us that had a wonderful guided prayer on it called "Anointing before Surgery," which I kept, of course.

They asked us to gather in a circle after Mass in front of the altar as they led this special prayer and anointing. Father Matthew

ACTION ITEMS

ACTION ITEMS

began the reading, we recited our parts, and then he blessed me with oil. After the prayer was finished everyone hugged me. Then, of course, I gave out my typed-up pink prayer sheets that reminded everyone to begin to pray for me thirty minutes prior to my surgery at 7:30 a.m. on Wednesday, June 10, the date of my surgery.

No matter your religion—Christianity, Judaism, Islam, Hinduism, Buddhism, or whatever—I found great comfort in my faith knowing that there is a force, a presence bigger than anyone on this planet who's got my back. You may feel the same—*pray*.

FINDING PEACE

As I continued to prepare myself for surgery and spoke with my anesthesiologist, got my healing statements written up, distributed my prayer sheets to all, and had my blessing in church, I also worked on centering myself and calming my ever-growing anxiety. I listened to Huddleston's relaxation CDs almost daily leading up to my surgery. On the Johns Hopkins Breast Center website, I came across a practice called yoga nidra and a complimentary forty-minute video presented by the Hopkins Kimmel Cancer Center[16] (both of which I still listen to too this day). Yoga nidra is a guided meditation to induce full body relaxation and deep rest. The practice has been found to reduce symptoms of anxiety, posttraumatic stress disorder, chronic pain, and insomnia, and it helps quiet the mind as well. These CDs and video helped relieve my anxiety tremendously.

DOING WHATEVER MAKES YOU FEEL BETTER

In researching preparing for surgery, I came across the Pink Lotus Breast Center in California, where Angelina Jolie allowed her journey (in preparing for her surgery) to be documented. It was called "A Patient's Journey: Angelina Jolie," by Dr. Kristi Funk.[17] Here

Action Items

Action Items

she chronicled how she readied herself for breast surgery by doing everything from gathering data and information on procedures to preparing her body with supplements and various regimens. These, for her, I gather, *as you will do for yourself*, made her feel she was taking control of not only her diagnosis but also preparing her body for surgery and the healing she would need after.

So, for instance, there were various supplements suggested that one may start taking to help wound healing, starting with vitamin C. Or, to reduce postoperative swelling and bruising, an herb called arnica,[18] a genus of perennial, herbaceous plants in the sunflower family. Or bromelain,[19] a pineapple extract to reduce inflammation. Also, to help with the elimination of anesthesia from your system more quickly, milk thistle or Exchem[20]; or, to help minimize scarring she suggested Bio-Corneum.[21] For this, I used CICACARE gel sheets, which I found most effective as my scars healed wonderfully. And I researched and cross-referenced everything! I came across the healing properties of Manuka honey, marketed as having not only antibacterial properties at the medical grade level but also being helpful in treating cancer and systemic inflammation.[22]

Yes, there were articles on the other side of things that discussed supplements and medications you may need to *stop taking* prior to surgery. One article cited the need to avoid drinking alcohol one month prior to surgery to ensure your liver is operating optimally, as well as not taking acetaminophen; both of these are notably toxic to the liver. Importantly, whatever information you come across on various topics, you absolutely need to engage and discuss all with your doctor.

A tip I implemented from Ms. Jolie's excellent resource list for prep before surgery was washing with Hibiclens to reduce the risk of infection. Although it said to use this twenty-four hours prior

Action Items

Action Items

to surgery, I cleansed pretty much my entire body a couple of days before. It is sold over the counter. I also came across the following information on the Memorial Sloan Kettering Cancer website:

> Your healthcare team has recommended that you shower with Hibiclens. Hibiclens is a skin cleanser that kills germs for up to 24 hours after using it. It contains a strong antiseptic (liquid used to kill germs and bacteria) called chlorhexidine gluconate. Showering with Hibiclens will help reduce your risk of infection.[23]

MINI MENTION

So as I sat in my blue net cap and gown and booties waiting to be taken to the OR, a nurse came in and gave me a few "wipes" to clean myself. I'm like, "What are these for?" She told me, "It's an antibacterial."

Here again, just another example of learning about something at your appointment—albeit this a major surgery!—that no one tells you ahead of time! I thought, *How could a few wipes, used minutes before surgery, actually be effective in disinfecting my body versus properly preparing two days or twenty-four hours prior to surgery?* I did not use them as I felt I was already properly cleansed.

THE MENTAL AND EMOTIONAL BENEFITS OF PHYSICAL ACTIVITY

As I continued researching, I read how surgery takes a big toll on your body, and you need to get yourself into shape prior to surgery so that you can look forward to a speedier recovery and bouncing

ACTION ITEMS

ACTION ITEMS

back faster. I continued with my yoga classes, bike classes, swimming, and exercising with weights. I wanted to ensure I was strong and fit and had done everything to make sure I would come through surgery just fine! Lifting weights, while nothing too crazy heavy, helped build up my strength a little so that I'd be able to push and prop myself up in bed and eventually open those impossible-to-open medicine bottles. Keeping focused at the gym also helped me (a bit) to keep my mind off the impending surgery.

I won't say much more on how *you* may want to prepare for surgery to maximize and improve your recovery process, but there excellent and unlimited resources and steps you can look into on your own—and I know you will! I am not a clinician, and of course, with everything there are benefits and risks and individual health factors that come into play. As always, do your research, reach out to and consult your doctor and care team, and be prepared!

INSPIRATION CAN LIFT YOU AND GET YOU THROUGH IT

Flashback to my wonderful Parisian friend Christiane. While we were in different countries, at different stages of life, we now shared a bond even more strongly than the length of time (more than ten years) that we had known one another, even greater than our apartment swaps. We shared the same journey and understanding of both having had breast cancer.

While we had more than 3,500 miles between us, from Manhattan to Paris, Christiane, through our email exchanges, could no doubt sense the growing concern I had as surgery was now just three days away. I saved a wonderful email she sent me. She was so confident and inspiring. And she was convinced that I, like she, would in fact *wake up* from surgery, and that was greatly comforting. Here I share her very personal email as it may comfort *you*!

Action Items

Action Items

Thank you, dear Arlene, I was thinking about Lisieux.
The best for you is. . . . DO NOT THINK . . . just do
something you like.
Before my last operation I went to Museum Pompidou (I had
four in two years and don't remember about the others).
But then, you come back tired and fall asleep right away until
the next day. Then you take your suitcase and go to the hospital.
Walk if it's not too far . . .
There the team will take you in charge and everything will be simple.
You're young, healthy, there is no reason to be afraid; this man
knows his job and hundreds of women get that kind of surgery
every day.
Send me a messages when you wake up . . .
Love, Christiane

STAYING POSITIVE

Tuesday, June 9, 2015, just one day before surgery—The day before
my surgery, taking the advice of my good friend across the
pond, I just did "something I liked." And *you* will do the same.
Do something you like! So I stepped out of my apartment and
walked a few blocks over to the Museum of Natural History's
Hayden Planetarium and purchased my ticket for the show on
the universe. Of course, as I'm online, waiting to get in, the
nurse calls with a few final questions and pieces of information.
Healthcare—even major surgeries—always at the last minute!

THE UNIVERSE GIVES US WHAT WE NEED; WE JUST HAVE TO RECOGNIZE IT

Wednesday, June 10, 2015, my day of surgery—Praying, being
prayed for, exercising, keeping in close contact with my doctors,
meditating, and keeping myself grounded and centered . . . the

Action Items

Action Items

day of surgery went extremely smoothly, and there were *many* signs that I was, without question, being looked after from above.

As I was escorted by a nurse who was lovely (but whom I didn't know, and a bit cold) and started to walk into the OR in my blue net cap and gown and booties, I thought, *I guess they do this all the time.* Then I heard another clinician in the hallway say, "Nadia." How crazy was this? It was a nurse I had worked with at my thoracic conference back in March, which was the very same conference I worked on with the doctor who helped me, at a pivotal moment, in my journey. So as I saw her passing I said, "Nadia?" She looked at me, unsure who I was. Obviously, I figured I looked a bit different in a blue net cap, gown, and booties than in a blue business suit. I said, "It's Arlene." She said, "Oh yes, the project manager." I then felt a comfort with her there as she was someone I knew; I felt her warmth as I headed into this major surgery. When I asked if she was one of my nurses, she paused. I gathered she wasn't, but she never said no (likely to comfort me), and then she said, "Oh, let me gear up, and I'm coming in." She then literally and warmly grabbed me around my shoulders and scooped me up from the other nurse as the other nurse trailed now behind us. Honestly, what were the odds of meeting her there on that exact day at that exact moment?

As she continued to walk me toward a small, tight, cul-de-sac space of surgery suites, I looked up, and there above the entrance to the room where I was to have my surgery was the number fourteen. My birth date! I'm crying as I write this. *You too* will see your "signs" that will bring you great comfort, warmth, and a feeling of love around you. Just keep open and look for them!

In praying for weeks on end to have a smooth surgery, I prayed to a few favorite saints of mine, including St. Therese of

Action Items

Action Items

Lisieux, St. Michael, St. Joan, and too many more—all of whom I've always felt a strong presence and connection with. I prayed that all would be with me in that room on my day of surgery.

I prayed to Mary, the mother of Jesus, in particular, asking her to be present in the room and specifically requesting that she show her presence with her "blue hue" blessing us all, including myself, my surgeons, the anesthesiologist, and the entire team responsible for, yes, keeping me alive! Now for those of you who are not Catholic, in most depictions of Mary, she is in a blue cloak under a blue sky—thus, a blue hue. So as we continued to walk into the room, *immediately* standing out to me was, all around, a *blue hue*. How was this? Well, as I glanced around, quite frankly, it looked like 1970s blue bathroom tiles all around the perimeter of this very small space. And with extremely bright lights bouncing off the tiles, it created a blue hue on the ceiling! Truly, I then knew I'd be okay.

Now all my doctors, nurses, and staff were starting to gather in the room. Nadia asked if I wanted a warm blanket; I said yes, and she quickly placed a few over me. We were literally talking about the next 2016 conference as I was jabbering away, trying to keep my mind off the anesthesia that was now starting to take effect. And then, before you knew it, four to five hours later I woke up in the recovery area. So the surgery went, as they say, "without event." And thank you, God! I woke up!

And yet the signs kept coming that day! In planning for surgery, I had asked the nurse and team that if I needed to share a room (which I found out I did as my insurance did not cover a private room), could I please have the side by the window with a view. But I also knew that request would be a long shot. They said of course they would try, but they could not promise it. So after recovery I was moved into my room

Action Items

Action Items

and there—*voila!*—was the empty bed right beside the window. Yes!

That evening I had a lot of pain and discomfort. In getting up to use the restroom I was having some trouble, and this lovely lady in the bed next to me said, "Can I help you?" I found out her name was Nancy. *How wonderful*, I thought, *that she offered me help*, but she was much older and looked like she might need help herself. So I told her to please not get up, that I was okay. But as she saw me struggling, she got out of her bed and helped me walk back to mine. Now it was quite late, after 10 p.m. Yet she started speaking with me and shared this was the second time she was in the hospital, that she was still recovering from sepsis.

She asked me what I was there for, and I told her breast surgery. She went on to tell me that thirty-seven years earlier, she had a mastectomy of her left breast and had an implant and it still looked great. Like, *really!* What were the odds of that, meeting someone in the same room who had breast cancer, who, too, could relate to and console me? Nancy shared that while she did have a lymph node that was positive and needed some chemo, she told me she was now eighty-two and doing great. She said, "My God, everyone has breast cancer," as she shared with me her sister-in-law had a double mastectomy. Although I was still heavily sedated and not completely lucid, I remember thinking that I just didn't think I'd ever not be surprised by the *staggering* numbers of women I was coming to find with breast cancer. So we chatted a bit more, and as it was getting late, Nancy said, "Okay, I'll put the light out soon, just after I say my prayer to Jesus and Mary."

Once more, I thought of the many signs I believe God had given me throughout this day:

ACTION ITEMS

ACTION ITEMS

- Blessing me with amazing surgeons and a surgical team

- Comforting me with someone I knew while walking into the OR, Nadia

- Seeing the number fourteen, my birth date, above the room I was to have surgery

- Mary's blue hue and knowing I was covered in love

- My room with a window view

- Gracing me with a roommate who was kind, comforting, and could relate to me as a woman who had had a breast removed and, thirty-seven years later, was doing great. *And she prays!*

And then there was the Eucharistic minister! *And here is that story.*

The next day, Nancy and I started to talk through the curtain a bit. Nancy came on over and sat by my bed. The conversation ranged about, and we were talking about religion. She showed me her cross and the medal of Mary she wore around her neck and said she had a special affection for Padre Pio. I shared with Nancy that I had gone to Lourdes in France. (Lourdes is where the Blessed Mother Mary appeared to St. Bernadette,[24] and it is here where millions pilgrimage daily for hope and healing. What a very special time it was for me there.) I shared with her that I too have a few favorite saints, among them St. Therese the Little Flower, and had visited Lisieux in Normandy in France where a basilica was built in her honor and where she grew up. And many more. (A few weeks later, after we had exchanged addresses and phone numbers, I printed out copies of photos and information on each site and mailed her hard copies in the mail.)

Action Items

Action Items

As we continued to talk about religion and our experiences, Nancy shared how disappointed she was that over the course of her hospital stay she hadn't been able to receive communion. It was at this *exact* moment (literally) that a woman walked into the room and said, "Hi, my name is Bettina, and I'm a Eucharistic minister and wanted to know if you would like to receive communion." *Really!* Bettina also sat and talked with us for about thirty minutes. She was lovely. And by the way, as I'm always sensitive to names and their meaning, I looked up what the name "Bettina" means. Here it is—*Bettina is a female name predominantly found in the Italian and German languages. . . . Benedetta is the Italian feminine form of Benedict, meaning "Blessed."* God is always at work!

> "For where two or three gather in my name, there am I with them."
>
> —*Jesus*[25]

ACTION ITEMS

ACTION ITEMS

NOTES

"I do not feel any less of a woman.
I feel empowered that I made
a strong choice that in no way
diminishes my femininity."

—*Angelina Jolie*[1]

Chapter Seven
Recovery: Landmark Firsts and Things You're Too Embarrassed to Ask

I f you are someone who wants to know more candid details post-surgery, then read on! Much of what I address in this chapter I found out on my own and wasn't fully prepared to handle. I want to share some things so you may be better prepared to address them. I keep upbeat and positive because what other option do we have? Right! We are survivors! With that said, the emotions and overall experience through this have been overwhelming, yet I feel extremely blessed—*as you will be too*—in meeting those breast friends who will guide you along your journey step-by-step.

As I chose breast reconstruction, in this chapter I'll give you a rundown on the unfolding of all three surgeries that it took to put me back together again and what each one accomplished, leading to that final step: the tattoo! Keep in mind that each journey is unique. There are myriad breast reconstruction options available today, and there is no one-size-fits-all. Which procedure you choose may vary based on your diagnosis or preference. Some of you may choose or have chosen implants, others a flap or tissue transfer, and yet others no reconstruction at all.

Initially, not sure how personal I wanted to get in this chapter, I quickly thought of those breast friends who shared their most intimate and personal details with me—someone they didn't know at all—so openly to help me prepare for what was ahead. So no matter who knews, firsts, or things that might be embarrassing to talk about, to honor those who came before me and their courage and unwavering support, here in this chapter, I'm putting it all out there. So let's get started!

When I was prepping for surgery, there was one breast friend in particular who instinctively knew that I had *intimate and personal* questions whirling around in my mind. It was on our second phone call together that it was like she read my mind and came right out sharing answers to those exact questions I had—questions I wanted to ask but felt too embarrassed to ask. For instance, while there was no clinical reason to remove her left breast—her MRIs were clean, she did not have the BRCA gene, and her mammograms showed normal (these were the exact same for me too)—the option was still made available to her, as it was to me as well. However, she reasoned and chose not to have a mastectomy of her left breast because, as she shared with me unabashedly, she wanted to be able to still feel that sexual stimulation on her real breast and nipple. Having had my breast friends' guidance, I was able to better think through and best assess all my options. I'm *so grateful* she spoke with me so candidly, as that in part is how this chapter came about.

Post-surgery I came to realize certain daily tasks that prior to surgery were effortless were now most difficult. You may have a quicker and easier recovery. My body needed months to regain

ACTION ITEMS

ACTION ITEMS

its strength and agility. It was then that the "who knews" and "firsts" started to pile up, along with all those simple tasks I had to learn to do again. Like, who knew I wouldn't have the strength to prop myself up in bed or open those impossible-to-open medication bottles? Like, the first time after surgery I was able to take a shower *with the lights on,* as I was too afraid to look down—and you may be too. And that's okay! The first time my physical therapist made me touch "it"—my new breast—it was weird. It felt weird and was scary looking. No—it was *frightening*!

Knowing I would be out of commission after surgery, I did my best the week before to get my hair done and a mani-pedi. I felt that if I was going to be in the hospital, I wanted to look and go in feeling the absolute best I could . . . or at least not completely disheveled. Make sure to do as much as possible before your surgery, ask for help ahead of time, and make sure your home is ready for your arrival. Be prepared!

THREE SURGERIES

The first surgery was in early June. During this surgery I had a mastectomy of my right breast. I chose not to remove my left breast because the MRI and all tests showed no DCIS or cancer. Top of mind was what my breast friend shared with me and her reasoning for not removing her left breast.

With that, they removed my right breast and placed in a tissue expander, and I opted for a silicone breast implant on the opposite side. A tissue expander is an empty breast implant that will be filled with normal saline over six to eight weeks. This process slowly stretches your skin and pectoralis muscle (large muscle in your chest). When your expander reaches the size your surgeon and you agree on, they stop the expansion process.

Action Items

Action Items

It was during this first surgery that they removed lymph nodes to test if the DCIS had spread, and they removed all the breast tissue to test for other cancer. It was after this they found I actually had an invasive cancer, staged at 1A. Remember: biopsies do not always tell the full story. They pulled a small sampling of cells, and my two breast biopsies missed the small amount of invasive cancer that had already developed.

In addition, it was during this first surgery they placed a breast implant in my left breast to help create symmetry and, bottom line, make them look as even as possible. As I'm a very visual person and visualizing a mastectomy was a difficult concept to grasp, one doctor shared, "Think of it as if you are replacing the stuffing in a pillowcase." *Hm, okay.* Well, that did help a bit, I guess.

About four months later, in October, after the tissue expansion was finished, I had my second surgery to remove the tissue expander and place the actual breast implant. This was a one-day outpatient procedure where I checked into the hospital early in the morning and left to go home in the very late afternoon. Here you need to have someone with you. Anytime you receive anesthesia, you will need someone there with you to pick you up and make sure you get home safely.

In addition, post-surgery you will go home with a Jackson-Pratt (JP) drain, also called a JP Drain. You, a family member, or possibly a homecare nurse/caregiver can help you manage. I was told the drain would be with me for maybe a week or two. *Of course,* twenty-four very long and unexpected days later, it was removed. Regardless of your healing time, when you then visit your plastic surgeon, they will remove the drain right in their office.

ACTION ITEMS

ACTION ITEMS

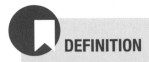

DEFINITION

JACKSON-PRATT (OR JP) DRAIN[2]

This is a closed-suction medical device that is commonly used as a postoperative drain for collecting bodily fluids from surgical sites. The drain itself is inside the body. The drain is connected to clear plastic tubing, which is usually sutured to the skin at the point it leaves the skin. The tubing connects to a bulb reservoir. The bulb, when squeezed empty, applies constant suction to the drain and pulls the fluid out of the body. The drain is removed when excess fluid has stopped draining from the body. Removal does not usually require an anesthetic. The purpose of a drain is to prevent fluid (blood or otherwise) buildup in a closed ("dead") space, as this may cause either disruption of the wound and the healing process or become an infected abscess, with either scenario possibly requiring a formal drainage/repair procedure (and possibly another trip to the operating room). If the drainage tubing becomes clogged or otherwise clotted off, the benefits are not realized in drainage.

Some people also may have their nipple removed. As mentioned in an earlier chapter, I wanted to take no chances of any cancer being left in my nipple. And as my BFF Hallia shared, "Why keep an old part on a new car?" I chose to have it removed. Thus, my third surgery (in late March 2016) was to reconstruct my nipple.

It just so happened that the day of my third surgery was also Good Friday, and I thought, *God will have my back. I'll be fine.* While the anxiety prior to each surgery diminished,

Action Items

Action Items

I never got fully comfortable with the idea of anesthesia, and there was always this underlying dread I would not wake up! But I did. *You too will be fine!* So this is the third and final surgery, when they create a nipple. I thought it would be the easiest and least impactful. While it was not especially painful per se, and while this surgery also was a one-day outpatient procedure (just one to two hours), it was still emotionally upsetting and devastating. When I looked down it was literally *frightening*—the stitches, the swelling . . . they made me feel sick when I looked. With that said, to prepare you, it heals beautifully!

Lastly, now more than a year after my first surgery, I got my areolar tattoo in late August 2016, making me whole again and completing breast reconstruction. If you choose to have this procedure, they will have you wait to ensure you are well healed. Timing is always different for everyone.

WHO KNEW? THE TATTOO

And finally, there's the areola, the darker-colored skin on your breast that surrounds your nipple. After seeing friends' tattoos through the years, I may have had a quick thought like, *Hm, if I was to get a tattoo, what would it be?* I first thought, *I love butterflies, so maybe a butterfly.* On a beach once, I noticed an inscription on a girl's arm, so I asked her what it meant. She said it was from the Bible and shared it was in Hebrew. It said, "There's a time to weep and a time to laugh, a time to mourn and a time to dance."[3] I thought, *How beautiful! Maybe?*

But I never thought in a gazillion years that the tattoo I'd actually end up getting in my lifetime was a tattoo of an areola on my right breast after three surgeries. Just sayin'! Also, once I decided to get the tattoo,

ACTION ITEMS

ACTION ITEMS

I quickly came to realize after speaking with many breast friends that getting a tattoo by a doctor was not the best route to go. Most women I spoke with shared the tattoo "faded quickly" or "it wasn't the right color" of their other areola or "the size was off" and so forth. I then thought, *Well I wouldn't go to a tattoo artist for breast surgery. Why would I go to a doctor for a tattoo?*

So I was off to find a real tattoo artist, one who could tattoo on my areola properly. That's when I found a *New York Times* online article titled "A Tattoo That Completes a New Breast."[4] It was an article showing women road tripping to Vinnie Myers's tattoo parlor[5] in Finksburg, Maryland. The article featured an amazing video that showed the work Myers and his team do to get women back together again so they can feel their best! But not wanting to head to Maryland, I started to search for tattoo artists in the geographic region where I lived. But I quickly came to find—which was hard to believe in Manhattan or even the surrounding regions—there was not one like Vinnie Myers's shop that was capable of this very specialized last and final step of breast reconstruction. So it was then that me and my BFF and gal pal Anita were off for a 422-mile roundtrip daytrip to Finksburg, Maryland.

WHO KNEW? YOU COULD ARGUE INSURANCE DECISIONS

Thus, after returning home with my new areola, I submitted my insurance claim, along with all appropriate documentation, to my health insurance company. My claim was denied. The insurance company said that Vinnie Myers, a specialized service, was not in my coverage. But they also shared there was not one healthcare provide or any tattoo artist who provided this service that could be covered in my health insurance plan. I thought, *How could this important finishing touch not be covered in your insurance?*

Action Items

Action Items

Thus, I was off to pay a visit to my breast surgeon. I explained to her how much I had to pay out of pocket and asked if she would be able to write a letter stating how important it was for me to have this covered and that it was in fact the last and final step in completing breast reconstructive surgery. She happily wrote the letter. The insurance company then told me to resubmit my claim along with my surgeon's letter. I did. This time my claim came back "processed" but *out-of-network,* which meant I'd have to meet my $1,000 deductible before I received any benefits. Thus, I got zero dollars from my $600 claim.

Then I thought, *It's not like I wanted to take a several hundred–mile road trip to another state, but with no providers in my geography, why not go to the best? And that was Vinnie Myers!* I once again called the insurance company, but this time I got the *right person* on the phone and now, almost seven months later, spoke with Alice. Alice, I could tell, *cared.* She listened intently to my story, and she was supportive—in short, she *got it, she understood.*

So after eight months of all-consuming, absolutely exhausting phone calls, emails, letters to my doctors, letters to the insurance company, and speaking with the insurance company, while $600 was not going to break my bank, I finally received full reimbursement. It was the *principle of the thing that kept me fighting.* How could a breast cancer patient who had breast reconstruction surgery not have access to *all* the right treatments to put herself back together to look whole again?

How could the insurance companies not have *any* provider, let alone an in-network provider, in one of the most densely populated regions in the United States, New York? Furthermore, given how common breast cancer is, how could any insurer not cover this service? My surgeon's office was a revolving door of breast patients, an extremely busy practice. Bottom line: keep pressing forward until you get *the right person* to hear you out, and *always* fight for what you feel is right.

Action Items

Action Items

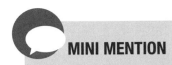

MINI MENTION

Let's address one of those things you may be too embarrassed to talk about.

Ladies, let me share: before your first surgery, your
plastic surgeon will ask you, "How big do you want to
go?" So here I am sitting on a table, down to the wire, days
before my surgery, and he's asking me about boob size.
Really! I'm completely freaked out about them removing
a body part, my breast of forty-nine years; going into a
four-hour surgery just hoping to wake up; stressing about
being out of work for several weeks; trying to remember
to prepare at my job, put my gym membership on hold,
and a gazillion other worries; and the last thing I felt I
could think about was the "inconsequential" question of
how big I wanted my new tatas to be!

Truth be told, once over the shock of such a personal
question—you'd think I'd be over all personal questions
by now!—well, since he asked, I did for a split-second
think, *Hm.* But I felt embarrassed to say, "Yes, doctor, I'd
like double Ds please." Okay, just kidding, that's too big.
But I did think, *A little bigger, maybe.* Instead, feeling awkward and embarrassed, I said, "Whatever is fine." Then I
recall mumbling something about "What do others do?"
God, it was mortifying! He said, to paraphrase, "Those
who choose to stay the same size often, after surgery, say
they wish they would have in fact gone one size bigger."

Anyway, point is, ladies: think about this beforehand.
What would I have done? I would have gone one size
bigger! Don't be shy.

Action Items

Action Items

WHO KNEW? YOU COULDN'T LIFT YOUR ARM

While everyone's recovery is very different, who knew—as no one shared with me—that after the first surgery, I wouldn't be able to do the simplest, most basic things like lift my arm to wash my hair?

Seven days after surgery, I headed to my hairdresser, Dina. At this point there was no way I could wash my own hair as I wasn't able to lift my right arm up at all, let alone over my head. Still, I wanted to start getting back to life as normal. At Dina's shop, even leaning back and positioning myself in Dina's chair was painful, but Dina, my fabulous hairdresser, eased me into it and . . . *voila!* My hair was washed and styled for the first time after surgery.

WHO KNEW? BLUE STOOL

As I've been asked by numerous women who too have been concerned and questioning after surgery why they may have delay in going to the bathroom[6] and/or *blue urine or stool,* here's why! The day prior to my surgery they told me they'd try to locate my lymph nodes by injecting a radioactive material[7] (depending on what time of day your surgery is, they may do this the same day), and after giving me two rounds of shots, the radioactive material was not moving to my lymph nodes as they wanted—*of course!* The idea was that the material would help them locate and remove the nodes during my surgery. I was told the next day—the day of my surgery—that instead of trying to get the radioactive material to work again, they would inject me with a blue dye—aha!—to help locate those nodes. Thus, post-surgery and five days later, alarmed my poo(!) was blue, I called my doctor, and she shared it was the dye. Relief! In a few different ways! To think, that dye was still in my body *five* days later. Make sure to drink a lot of fluids—especially water—to help your body eliminate toxins.

Action Items

Action Items

MY ELEVEN MOST IMPORTANT FIRSTS

1. **First Day Back in *My* Apartment**
   For seventeen days after surgery, I stayed with my mom and family. Having them to help me get through the early days was a huge blessing. It was not easy. *Thank you, Mom. I love you!* Think about who can help you on your recovery, short- or long-term. However long you need. Whether family, friends, colleagues or whoever, just reach out and ask!

2. **First *Specialized* Physical Therapy (PT) Appointment**
   As everyone is different and unique in their recovery, you may not even need PT. However, for me it was twenty-one days after surgery, two days before my JP drain came out, that I went for my first PT appointment with a therapist who specialized in breast cancer rehabilitation and lymphedema therapy.

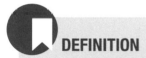

DEFINITION

LYMPHEDEMA THERAPY[8]
Treatment for lymphedema depends on the severity and extent of the condition.

Treatment options may include:

- **Exercise:** Exercise helps to restore flexibility and strength, and it improves drainage. Specific exercises will be recommended by your doctor and/or physical therapist.

- **Bandage:** Wearing a customized compression sleeve or elastic bandage may help to prevent an accumulation of fluid.

Action Items

Action Items

- **Arm pump:** Applying an arm pump often helps to increase the fluid flow in the lymphatic vessels and keeps fluid from collecting in the arm.

- **Diet:** Eating a well-balanced diet and controlling body weight is an important part of treatment.

- **Elevation:** Keeping the arm raised above the level of the heart, whenever possible, allows gravity to help drain the accumulated fluid.

- **Infection Prevention:** It is important to follow preventive measures, such as good skincare, to protect the affected arm from infection and skin breakdown.

I suggest you discuss this with your doctor, get recommendations, and get a first appointment lined up before your surgery. It's one less thing to think about as you're recovering. For me, after six months and forty sessions, I finally was able to move about more freely and lift my arm, almost over my head. Donna, my physical therapist, was an extraordinary clinician and a board-certified lymphedema therapist specializing in breast cancer rehabilitation. She was an amazing person. She not only helped me raise my arms up and move again, she raised my spirits.

As if there weren't enough awkward moments already on this journey, from baring your breasts to the plastic surgeon at that first consultation and looking at your new-to-be plastic boobs on his desk, now you have someone who's literally going to be seeing you topless when you don't look and feel your best and then touching and manipulating your new breast. It was while lying on her table during the first few

ACTION ITEMS

ACTION ITEMS

appointments, flat on my back, that she made me look down in the light and touch it! And I looked, for the first time, straight on at my new breast. She made me feel so comfortable. She listened intensely to my story, and I'm sure she must have heard endless similar stories over and over again. But she listened as if I was the only one who ever dealt with the issues that come after recovering from breast cancer surgery. Donna helped me recover both physically and emotionally. Donna, a simple message: I thank you from the bottom of my heart.

3. First Shower in the Dark

Twenty-two days after surgery, I finally took my first full shower. This, I have to tell you, was completely scary, and I spent the entire day contemplating how I was going to muster the courage to take that shower. Still having difficulty with arm movement and in pain, I was actually afraid to get the bandages wet. Frankly, while I did a tremendous amount of research preparing for this, I faint at the sight of blood, and I can't deal with cuts or anything of that nature. I still had that awful drain, and I didn't even know where the stitches were or where the incisions were made. I did not want a visual, and everything was numb anyway. It was a very difficult time. But I made it in the shower with my front-zip bra on and, slowly, was able to wash my hair for the first time myself and take my own shower. This was not easy. One more thing: I could not keep the lights on. I did not want to see anything. But I did glance down a little.

By the way, no one tells you to buy a front-zip bra![9] When you first leave the hospital, you have to figure it out. Ladies, please make sure you buy this before surgery. Then, when you come out of the bandages and dressings they put

Action Items

Action Items

around your chest when they send you on your way from the hospital, you will be prepared. And then, from home, you can transition at your own pace into the front-zip bra.

As your doctor will likely tell you, everything needs to stay tight; you need to wear this. Plus, you certainly will not be able to put on a regular bra. And, for sure, *no* under-wires. While this may sound silly, when shopping I literally had no clue what to buy. Be sure to look this up and buy a few front-zip bras before surgery.

4. First Visit to the Plastic Surgeon

Twenty-four days after surgery, and yes, after a record-setting twenty-four days going, the JP drain was *finally* removed. I call this record-setting as I was told it is usually removed anywhere from ten to twelve days after surgery. But of course, mine took twenty-four! I was calling the doctor's office incessantly: "Why is this taking so long?!" They told me, in so many words, that basically everyone's body is different and that mine just took longer. It is at the same doctor's appointment at which they remove the JP drain that they then expand the expander, snipping it out and then putting in a stitch or two where the point of entry was. *Arrgh! Cringe.* Then they are on to expanding the expander.

Not knowing what to expect as I was lying on the table, the doctor came up with a *very* long, thick needle with a *very* big barrel, and I was like, "What are you doing with that?" He calmly said—I'm sure my reaction was the same (or at least similar) to most when they first see it—that there was a magnet guide on the expander that directs the needle to the proper place to insert the saline. They do this over the course of several visits; the number of visits will depend on which size breast you chose.

Action Items

Action Items

As the saline is injected in, *get ready*! This literally felt like cinderblocks were being placed on my chest. I felt tremendous pressure in my chest, and it hurt to breathe. I was afraid to breathe, as something felt like it would break, but be assured nothing did, or does, and, like everything else, I survived! And you will too! Know this is the process you must go through to expand the space behind your chest wall with this temporary saline implant to make room for the actual and final and *real* breast implant that is inserted during the second surgery months later after things have healed a bit more. So, for me, about five days later, going back for the second expansion, this heavy, scary pressure happened once more as the doctor inserted more saline fluid.

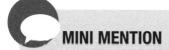

MINI MENTION

For those of you who choose not to have reconstruction, here's what Fiona, another breast friend, a longtime colleague and now very dear friend wanted me to share with you

After consulting with my breast surgeon and praying for guidance, I felt the best option for me was not to undergo reconstruction. I felt it was less invasive and I could get back to life sooner as I would only need one surgery. I would, however, be fitted for a prothesis, which was a simulated breast that would slip into a pocket in my bra or swimsuit. It's a decision that took some time to get accustomed to and one of the challenges I faced was that I had to find garments that were less revealing, being concerned that somehow if I bent over someone might be able to see more than I wanted them to. As an

Action Items

Action Items

eighteen-year survivor, I know in my heart it was the right decision for me.

5. First Time Rolling on to My Left Side and Sleeping in My Bed

Twenty-eight days after surgery—after sleeping on my back, propped up on pillows and blankets, initially at my mom's and then on my couch, for weeks—lying flat on a bed was painful and uncomfortable. It was after all this time that I stretched for the first time and was able to roll on my left side and sleep in my own bed. Gosh, it felt good to stretch and roll over!

6. First Time Food Shopping

Thirty days after surgery, I was able to get a little food shopping done. Again, shop ahead for food get as much as you can done in advance. While I had to adjust to the fact that I could not be lifting heavy bags like I used to, I did manage to get some fresh produce and pick up some items for the weekend. Less is more going forward.

7. First Time Doing My Own Laundry

Thirty-one days after surgery, with a little help from my friend and neighbor, I was able to get over to the laundromat a few blocks away. It was a small load, but I needed to get it done. My neighbor carried it to and from, and I was able to get it in the washing machine and dryer. Halleluiah! I love to do my own laundry, so this was great. It makes you feel like life is getting back to normal.

ACTION ITEMS

ACTION ITEMS

8. First Time I Kinda Felt Like … Myself

Nearly five weeks after surgery—in early July—I noted I finally felt like myself. I felt my strength coming back. I didn't feel lethargic. I was drinking a ton of water trying to flush out all the anesthesia they say lingers in your body for weeks. I was taking my vitamins and recovering slowly, one day at a time. I was *patient* with my Type A self. So allow me the liberty of some quick text-speak: XoXoXo. Be patient with yourself too!

9. First Shower with the Light *On*

Five weeks after surgery—now mid-July—I knew I'd be headed back to work the next week and was now feeling a bit better, stronger. So I took my first shower with the lights *on*. For me, as it may be for you, it was brutal seeing the scarring and stitches, which were still dissolving. *Brutal.* It was in this shower that, also for the first time, I shaved my armpits and legs. Also, I scheduled a mani-pedi with Maria at my nail salon. Life does get back to normal; it did for me and *will for you too! Be patient with yourself!*

10. First Day Back to Work

Six weeks after surgery, now late July, was my first day back to work. Ladies, while I had initially thought, *Oh, four weeks will be fine*, everyone's recovery time and level of tolerance for pain is different! So please trust me here. If you can take the time off, *take all the time you can* away from work to recover as best and as fully as you can.

11. First Time Back to the Gym, and Yoga

Twelve weeks after surgery, now mid–September, for the first time I headed to the gym and took a yoga class with Suzanne.

Action Items

Action Items

Now I was not just celebrating one day during the year, my birthday, but back to and celebrating life *every single day*!

FINAL PATHOLOGY

Two weeks after surgery, after appointments with my breast surgeon and plastic surgeon, thankfully I received good news. The final pathology came back and was negative for cancer in all three lymph nodes. It was, however, positive for 3.5 millimeters of invasive cancer, which then staged me at Stage 1A breast cancer. I was told this was "far" from any margins, so that was okay. And while I was told that I likely would not need chemotherapy or radiation, my breast surgeon had me follow up and see a medical and radiation oncologist.

Also, it was at this one appointment my breast surgeon and I joked that she won the Tamoxifen battle! While I told her, initially, "I will not take a pill every day for five years," post-surgery, after researching the benefits and risks of Tamoxifen and learning that cancer feeds off estrogen, it was clear the benefits *for me* far outweighed the risks. I recalled telling the doctor "I won't take it," and her saying, "Yes, you will." She was right!

I took my first Tamoxifen pill on my fiftieth birthday, August 14, 2015, and I completed my five years of Tamoxifen on August 14, 2020! Time flew for me, and it will too for you!

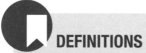

DEFINITIONS

SURGICAL MARGIN[10]
The surgeon's goal during surgery is to take out all the breast cancer along with a rim of normal tissue around it.

ACTION ITEMS

ACTION ITEMS

This is to be sure all the cancer has been removed. During or after surgery, a pathologist examines this rim of tissue—called the **surgical margin** or **margin of resection**—to be sure it's clear of any cancer cells. If cancer cells are present, this will influence decisions about treatments, such as additional surgery and radiation. Margins are checked after surgical biopsy, lumpectomy, and mastectomy.

CLEAR (ALSO CALLED NEGATIVE OR CLEAN)

No cancer cells are seen at the outer edge of the tissue removed. Sometimes the pathology report will tell you the width of the "clear margin": the distance between the outer edge of the surrounding tissue removed and the edge of the cancer. When margins are clear, usually no additional surgery is needed.

POSITIVE

Cancer cells come out to the edge of the removed tissue. More surgery is usually needed to remove any remaining cancer cells.

CLOSE

Cancer cells are close to the edge of the tissue but not right at the edge. More surgery may be needed.

An important note: There is not a standard definition of how wide a "clear margin" has to be. In some hospitals, doctors want 2 millimeters or more of normal tissue between the edge of the cancer and the outer edge of the removed tissue. In other hospitals, however, doctors

Action Items

Action Items

consider a 1 mm rim of healthy tissue—and sometimes even smaller than that—to be a clear margin. As you talk with your doctor about whether your margins were clear, positive, or close, you also can ask how "clear" is defined by your medical team.

TAMOXIFEN AND UTERINE/ENDOMETRIAL CANCER

Tamoxifen[11] is a drug used to treat certain types of breast cancer in women and men. It is also used to prevent breast cancer in women who have had ductal carcinoma in situ (DCIS, abnormal cells in the ducts of the breast) and in women who are at a high risk of developing breast cancer. Tamoxifen is a type of endocrine therapy and blocks the effects of the hormone estrogen in the breast. Tamoxifen is a type of antiestrogen. It is being studied for use with other types of cancer as well. Tamoxifen is typically taken daily by mouth for five years for breast cancer.

While Tamoxifen acts as an antiestrogen in breast tissue, it acts like an estrogen in the uterus. In women who have gone through menopause, it can cause the uterine lining to grow, and this increases the risk of endometrial cancer.

The risk of developing endometrial cancer from Tamoxifen is low (less than 1 percent per year). Endometrial cancer is a type of cancer that begins in the uterus. Most uterine cancers begin in the lining of the uterus, which is called the endometrium. Endometrial cancer is sometimes called uterine cancer.

Uterine (endometrial) cancer is the most common cancer of the female reproductive system with more than

ACTION ITEMS

ACTION ITEMS

49,500 American women diagnosed with the disease each year.[12] It tends to develop after menopause when a woman is between the ages of 50 and 60.

MY VISIT WITH THE MEDICAL ONCOLOGIST

It was about three weeks after surgery that I first met the oncologist. Thankfully, it was all good except for the confirmation that they did find a very small amount—3.5 millimeters—of invasive cancer. But all of that was removed.

All other markers that he discussed, like estrogen and progesterone, were positive, which is good, and "HER2" was negative. He said, "This is a great thing," as hormone receptor-positive breast cancer accounts for about 80 percent of all breast cancers[13] and is called "ER-positive." That means the cancer cells grow in response to the hormone estrogen. About 65 percent of these are also "PR-positive."[14] They grow in response to the hormone progesterone. If your breast cancer has a significant number of receptors for either estrogen or progesterone, it is considered hormone-receptor positive. Thus, tumors that are ER/PR-positive have a good prognosis because they can benefit from endocrine therapy.

 DEFINITIONS

The ovaries maintain the health of the female reproductive system. They secrete two main hormones: **estrogen**[15] and **progesterone**.[16]

Action Items

Action Items

Estrogens are hormones that are important for sexual and reproductive development, mainly in women. They are also referred to as female sex hormones. The term *estrogen* refers to all of the chemically similar hormones in this group, which are **estrone**, **estradiol** (primary in women of reproductive age), and **estriol**.

Progesterone is a female steroid sex hormone secreted by the corpus luteum to prepare the endometrium for implantation, and later by the placenta during pregnancy, to prevent rejection of the developing embryo or fetus.

You may have hormone therapy after surgery, chemotherapy, and radiation are finished. These treatments can help prevent a return of the disease by blocking the effects of estrogen and, while there are several ways to do this treatment, one, as I wrote above, is a medication called Tamoxifen (also called Nolvadex), which helps stop cancer from coming back by blocking hormone receptors and thus preventing hormones from binding to them. It's sometimes taken for as many as five years after initial treatment for breast cancer. In HER2-positive breast cancer, which is about 20 percent of breast cancers, the cells make too much of a protein known as HER2. These cancers tend to be aggressive and fast-growing.

At my visit the oncologist also talked about possibilities of recurrence and taking what's called the Oncotype DX.[17] I did take the Oncotype DX test about four weeks after my first visit. It tests your own tumor's genes to determine your risk of recurrence with or without chemotherapy or endocrine therapy. This can be costly, and as I've shared in earlier chapters, you should make sure that your insurance company covers this test, and if so, always get your authorization in writing.

Action Items

Action Items

It turned out, as the doctor reported, that according to the Oncotype DX, that my cancer was "negative for aggressive disease" and, with taking Tamoxifen for five years, my risk factor of recurrence after ten years was under 10 percent. And I had no need for chemotherapy. I digress in mentioning that, the day after my first meeting with the oncologist, the radiation oncologist also confirmed good news: there was no need for radiation.

 MINI MENTION

As our treatment and our options are most unique to our diagnosis, below my beautiful, most awesome, breast friend Fiona shared with me her experience to help guide and inspire those of you who are reading this and may need radiation and or chemotherapy. She's a positive force, and I'm so blessed to know her and have her in my life, and her words will no doubt resonate with you and give you hope:

After my pathology report was reviewed by my oncologist, it was determined I had stage III breast cancer and some lymph node involvement. I asked my doctor if lymph node involvement meant my survival odds were lower and he said, "Everyone is different," and assured me he would do everything to help me.

It did mean I had to go through a few months of chemo followed by radiation treatment. How would I get through this? I made a plan because it made me feel in control. For example, who would come with me to treatments, what I could do during the treatments, and

Action Items

Action Items

how I would reward myself after treatments. I also went to see a complementary medicine clinician who gave me the best advice: "The best medicine is to surround yourself with those you love and to laugh daily."

Well, the day my young children took turns wearing my wig had me in tears of laughter and created a memory I could hold on to and use whenever I needed it most. He couldn't have been more right. I also kept myself busy and never dwelled on my condition. Having a positive attitude is key to recovery. So through about nine months of challenges, today I am here to let you know you can be a survivor too.

MY VISIT WITH THE RADIATION ONCOLOGIST

In early July I met with the radiation oncologist. The funny thing is that my breast surgeon, at our last meeting, gave me a card to contact the radiation oncologist and make an appointment. Looking down at the business card, I realized this was a doctor I knew well as I had worked with him before managing a continuing medical education conference for him.

When I met with him, he was amazingly positive. He said there was no need for any radiation. Still conflicted, even post-surgery, meeting with him for the first time, I shared my struggle with DCIS as to whether it should be considered "real cancer" or not. And *he* was the one I had always been searching for, to give the answer I was yearning to hear: "Arlene, this is not cancer." I never had one doctor even hint at this (well, kind of—my primary care hinted at no need for treatment on the level of getting a mastectomy), but it was the radiation oncologist who

ACTION ITEMS

ACTION ITEMS

said, "This is not cancer." And, thankfully, I never found that person (to say what I was looking for) *pre*-surgery as, remember, it had already turned into invasive cancer, and it was my decision, based on extensive research and information, my doctors, and breast friends' experiences, that I chose to have surgery. And thank God I did.

HEALING AND THE FUTURE

I continue to have an outstanding group of healthcare providers (as you will too as they are with us for our lifetime) from the amazing front desk team who book our appointments and get our test authorizations to my breast surgeon, oncologist, and my gynecologist, all of whom I now see once a year for annual checkups. We must be diligent in our checkups and self-care.

Also now added to my list of annual checkups are my new doctors who are part of the 9/11 World Trade Center (WTC) Health Program.[18] As I shared in an earlier chapter, having worked at the New York Stock Exchange on 9/11 and four years after, as most of my journey has been, simply by pure chance it was that one day I was talking with a colleague and good friend, Francine, that I learned about this program. And after applying, I received notification that I was certified and enrolled as a certified-eligible survivor, making me eligible for lifetime monitoring and treatment benefits for the listed certified health condition, breast cancer.

Furthermore, if you lived at, worked at, or helped with the rebuilding in the Ground Zero zone during 9/11 and developed cancer or a host of diseases, you should make sure to visit the 9/11 WTC Health Program and 9/11 Victim Compensation Fund[19] websites.

Action Items

Action Items

DEFINITIONS

9/11 WTC HEALTH PROGRAM

The WTC Health Program offers high-quality, compassionate care to those directly affected by the September 11 terrorist attacks in New York, the Pentagon, and in Shanksville, Pennsylvania. Members of the WTC Health Program share a common experience—they were present during the days and months following the terrorist attacks of September 11, 2001. From that common experience, members have their own unique story. Some worked long hours during the rescue, recovery, and cleanup efforts. Others returned to their homes, businesses, and schools in lower Manhattan. Today many of them confront 9/11-related health issues such as asthma, GERD, post-traumatic stress, even cancer.

9/11 VICTIM COMPENSATIONS FUND

The September 11th Victim Compensation Fund was created to provide compensation for any individual (or a personal representative of a deceased individual) who suffered physical harm or was killed as a result of the terrorist-related aircraft crashes of September 11, 2001, or the debris removal efforts that took place in the immediate aftermath of those crashes.

"The race on the beach renews ones youth like a dip in the sea. But we are no longer children, life is not a beach. There is no pattern here for permanent return, only for refreshment."

—*Anne Morrow Lindbergh*

NOTES

"Own your diagnosis and
don't let it own you!"

—*Arlene M. Karole, CHCP*

Chapter Eight
Ductal Carcinoma in Situ (DCIS): How Do You Define Cancer?
Is It or Isn't It?

I include this very brief chapter on ductal carcinoma in situ, or DCIS, as on my journey, I came across alarming and also seemingly conflicting information on what DCIS is and how to treat it. This led to some confusion as to what I should do given my diagnosis. I am including this brief chapter for you who may come across some of the very same literature and information I did. Overall, DCIS represents close to 20 percent of breast cancers detected by screening every year.[1]

When I first started researching DCIS, this came up: "The National Institutes of Health estimates that by 2020, more than 1 million women in the U.S. will be living with a DCIS diagnosis" along with the NIH State-of-the-Science Conference Statement on "Diagnosis and Management of Ductal Carcinoma in Situ" from September 2009.[2] Needless to say, this was an incredibly huge number. My next and immediate thought was, if my diagnosis of DCIS was initially missed by my two mammograms and one ultrasound, how can it be caught? Noted in that NIH conference statement:

> As of January 1, 2005, an estimated one-half-million U.S. women were living with a diagnosis of DCIS. The prevalence is greater in white women than in black women and women of other races and/or ethnicities. If we assume constant incidence and survival rates, it is estimated that by 2020 more than 1 million living U.S. women will have a diagnosis of DCIS.

That same conference went on to say:

> Ductal carcinoma in situ of the breast, or DCIS, represents a spectrum of abnormal cells confined to the breast duct and is a risk factor for invasive breast cancer development. Unlike invasive breast cancer, DCIS either has not yet invaded beyond its intraductal origin or may never invade neighboring tissues. DCIS is most often diagnosed as a consequence of screening for invasive breast cancer because DCIS has no specific screening modality. The etiology of DCIS is presumably heterogeneous, making assessment of prognosis based on pathology and imaging highly variable. On the basis of pathological and molecular studies, some DCIS represents a precursor to invasive breast cancer; *however, the proportion of untreated DCIS that will progress to invasive breast cancer is unknown.*

The diagnosis and management of DCIS is highly complex with many unanswered questions, including the fundamental natural history of untreated disease. *Because of the noninvasive nature of DCIS, coupled with its favorable*

ACTION ITEMS

ACTION ITEMS

prognosis, strong consideration should be given to remove the anxiety-producing term "carcinoma" from the description of DCIS. The outcomes in women treated with available therapies are excellent. Thus, the primary question for future research must focus on the accurate identification of patient subsets diagnosed with DCIS, including those persons who may be managed with less therapeutic intervention without sacrificing the excellent outcomes presently achieved. Essential in this quest will be the development and validation of accurate risk stratification methods based on a comprehensive understanding of the clinical, radiological, pathological, and biological factors associated with DCIS.

One sentence struck me: *"the proportion of untreated DCIS that will progress to invasive breast cancer is unknown."* That lead me to some confusion. I found myself asking, "Will my DCIS stay 'in situ,' or will it suddenly become invasive without me even realizing it?" And the next question "Do I really need to remove my breast, or can I just let it be?"

I was further confused by the following paragraph's second sentence—*"Because of the noninvasive nature of DCIS, coupled with its favorable prognosis, strong consideration should be given to remove the anxiety-producing term "carcinoma" from the description of DCIS."* At that time, I didn't know exactly what *carcinoma* meant (as I never had breast or any cancer before), and after looking it up, I realized it means cancer! So while I was somewhat relieved at this positive statement, noting some excellent outcomes and favorable prognosis of women diagnosed with DCIS, this led to some more confusion and another—perhaps the hardest—question: Is DCIS cancer or not?

Action Items

Action Items

As I continued on in my search for answers *to those questions*, I came across professionals within the medical community who had talked about a less aggressive approach to treating DCIS. Medically speaking, they proposed "active surveillance," and monitoring me with frequent breast imaging. In other words, doing nothing for now. Some doctors are seeking to rename and remove the "C" in DCIS, taking the approach more along the lines with the NIH conference statement and strongly considering removing the word *carcinoma* from the nomenclature. On the other hand, there are those clinicians taking a more aggressive approach to treatment, saying I should consider something more radical than seemingly necessary (like a double mastectomy).

Here again I am reminded of that *Time* magazine article I read in October 2015, just months after my mastectomy. It addressed that very question—"How much is too much?"—with the cover article titled "What if I Decide to Just Do Nothing?"

At first glance at that magazine cover, I felt a deeply sickening feeling and questioned my decision. Should I have *not had* a mastectomy? Did I make the right choice? I thought, *Yes, for me it was. I absolutely made the right choice*, since it turned out my DCIS had already turned into invasive cancer. It was only after my surgery that the pathology came back, and I was then diagnosed with Stage 1A cancer. Thankfully I had already taken action and did not wait and see.

With that, in this article a prominent doctor on the West Coast, Dr. Laura Esserman, a surgeon and the director of the Carol Franc Buck Breast Care Center at the University of California, San Francisco (UCSF) notes, "If we were doing so well and no one was dying, I would agree we don't need to change. But patients don't like the treatment options, and physicians don't like the outcomes."[3] The article goes on to note that

ACTION ITEMS

ACTION ITEMS

Esserman, along with Dr. Shelley Hwang, professor of surgery and chief of breast surgical oncology at the Duke University School of Medicine in Durham, North Carolina, are leading a number of studies that they hope will fill in some of the knowledge gaps that make change such an uphill battle.[4]

Dr. Esserman is creating a DCIS registry at the five University of California Medical Centers. Women diagnosed with DCIS at any of the facilities will be offered options including active surveillance and being tracked over time.[5] This article has some interesting and insightful information from several perspectives from doctors and patients.

I also came across an interview with Dr. Shelley Hwang from the 2017 San Antonio Breast Cancer Symposium (SABCS) titled "'Cultural Change': Dialing Back the Discussion and Treatment of DCIS."[6] This is a video you don't want to miss.

Further adding to my hesitancy of having a mastectomy as I shared earlier in this book, after meeting with several breast surgeons I was told by one that DCIS is an "excellent diagnosis and is 99 percent curable" and by another it was a "miracle" that it was found (remember ladies, trust your gut and persist if you feel something isn't right—it may not be!). So, again, it sounded like great news to hear, but I just couldn't grasp then why such a drastic treatment as a mastectomy, a removal of a body part that I'd had for forty-nine years!

Furthermore, in my research I came across the below paper on DCIS. Basically, it notes that while virtually all invasive cancer begins as DCIS, not all DCIS will go on to become invasive. I realized there is seemingly no scientific evidence available, at least at this point in time, assuring and guaranteeing us which cells will and won't change to invasive cancer, and that's why

Action Items

Action Items

DCIS is treated as cancer even if the jury may be out on whether or not we should actually *call* it cancer.

In *Critical Reviews™ in Eukaryotic Gene Expression*, volume 24, issue 4, this published paper titled "Ductal Carcinoma in Situ: A Brief Review of Treatment Variation and Impacts on Patients and Society" says:

> Nearly 20% of all breast cancer cases are ductal carcinoma in situ (DCIS), with over 60,000 cases diagnosed each year. Many of these cases would never cause clinical symptoms or threaten the life of the woman; however, it is currently impossible to distinguish which lesions will progress to invasive disease from those that will not. DCIS is generally associated with an excellent prognosis regardless of the treatment pathway, but there is variation in treatment aggressiveness that seems to exceed the medical uncertainty associated with DCIS management. Therefore, it would seem that a significant proportion of women with DCIS receive more extensive treatment than is needed. This overtreatment of DCIS is a growing concern among the breast cancer community and has implications for both the patient (via adverse treatment-related effects, as well as out-of-pocket costs) and society (via economic costs and the public health and environmental harm resulting from health care delivery).[7]

Regardless, across the board, all doctors I met with agreed with the extensive amount of DCIS that was found with the two breast needle biopsies, documented between eight to nine centimeters in my right breast, and they alluded to it was not if, *but when* the DCIS would turn to invasive cancer. Not one doctor said, "Do not get a mastectomy." Bottom line: doctors

ACTION ITEMS

ACTION ITEMS

will likely not deviate from what's called the *standard of care*. As noted in that *Time* article, "They may face malpractice lawsuits and doctors do not want to be responsible for the patient who isn't treated aggressively and dies on their watch."[8] When I looked up the current standard treatment for DCIS, it was a lumpectomy followed by radiation or mastectomy.[9]

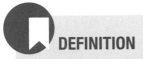

DEFINITION

STANDARD OF CARE[10]

Standard of care is a diagnostic and treatment process that a clinician should follow for a certain type of patient, illness, or clinical circumstance, usually defined by a medical board in that specialty. In legal terms, the level at which the average, prudent provider in a given community would practice. It is how similarly qualified practitioners would manage the patient's care under the same or similar circumstances. [A] medical malpractice plaintiff must establish the appropriate standard of care and demonstrate that the standard of care has been breached.

While there were a couple of surgical options available to me, I also had the option to keep an eye on it and wait with surveillance and biopsies every three to six months. But I thought for me, that was not the approach I wanted to take. I, like most breast friends I spoke with, just wanted "it" out of my body. I didn't feel active surveillance of this disease present in my body would give me the peace of mind that I needed to have. I was terrified to think about waiting and then to hear ultimately

Action Items

Action Items

it had spread to my lymph nodes or other organs. I did have choices, and *for me*, I was going to have a mastectomy.

With that said, it was not an easy decision. But it was a well-thought-out and an informed one! *And you too will need to do what's best for you!* You need to not only listen to your gut—as it was that little feeling of a simple *pinprick* on my right breast that made me question—you must also pay attention to your unique signs and symptoms[11] that may show with breast cancer (or *may not,* as that pinprick I felt wasn't noted on any list of signs to look for). Whether a change in the size, shape, or appearance of a breast, a newly inverted nipple,[12] or other symptoms, *pay attention* and seek medical advice!

"We need to be willing to let our intuition guide us, and then be willing to follow that guidance directly and fearlessly."

—*Shakti Gawain*[13]

ACTION ITEMS

ACTION ITEMS

NOTES

"We must not cease from exploration. And at the end of all our exploring will be to arrive where we began and know the place for the very first time."

— *T. S. Eliot*[1]

Epilogue

As I mentioned earlier in this book, one of my favorite quotes is spoken by Glinda the Good Witch in *The Wizard of Oz*. After her exhausting journey through Oz, Dorothy finally finds an opportunity to get home to Kansas, but then the hot air balloon leaves without her. Surrounded by her faithful companions, Dorothy cries and pleads for it to come back. It's in that moment when Glinda appears, and Dorothy asks how she'll ever get home. Glinda gently tells her, "My dear, you've always had the power to get back home, but you had to learn it for yourself." The Scarecrow chimes in, "Well, that's so easy, we should have thought of that for you." But, as Glinda makes clear, Dorothy had to find it out for herself.

Having read my breast cancer journey, you likely understand that, like Dorothy, I had to find my own way through it. I couldn't hope to be rescued or hop on a magic hot air balloon. I highlight certain themes over and over in this book: *empowerment, choice, knowledge,* and *action.* Like Dorothy, people who receive a diagnosis of cancer must put in the work and not relegate or delegate our choices or our destiny to others. We must realize that we are in control; each of us has agency and the capacity to act. We must find our own way home.

In this book, I've shared all that I've learned about making empowered decisions after a diagnosis. Refer to the seven steps on how to own and take charge of your diagnosis. Reference the forms, checklists, and resources I've included in this book. Review the glossary and notes for further reference. Use this as a workbook. Take it to your medical appointments. Ask a lot of questions, and take a lot of notes. (We've left you space to do so on the bottom of each page and at the end of each chapter.)

My exploration—my adventures in Oz, if you will—took me way beyond my breast cancer diagnosis and forced me to look inward and learn more about myself, taught me to reprioritize what's really important in life, and—like Dorothy's adventures—brought amazing companions into my life.

I learned so much about myself, as there in nothing more gut-wrenching than to hear those three words: "You have cancer." I began to examine my lifestyle choices: my diet and nutrition, my exercise regimen, my environment, the way I carry myself throughout the day, and my daily routines. While I am a proud, self-proclaimed type A-er, assertive and a go-getter and a multitasking wizard, running from one project to the next, it was along this journey I had that lightbulb moment when I stopped and asked myself, "How have my *choices* over a lifetime impacted my health in either positive—or not so positive—ways?"

Cancer isn't the only thing that causes us to turn inward and take a careful look at our lives. Other illnesses, natural disasters, inequities, tragedies, and yes, global pandemics, can do the same. When the noise of life's "normal" distractions is silenced,

ACTION ITEMS

ACTION ITEMS

we ponder the meaning of life. We learn new things about ourselves, set new goals, shift our priorities, and gain wisdom.

If you've just been diagnosed, I want you to know that no matter what your stage of life or stage of breast cancer—whether DCIS Stage 0, Stage 1, Stage 2, Stage 3, or Stage 4—there are tremendous advancements in research, medicine, and science that will help you. There are outstanding, evidence-based studies and information showing the positive outcomes and results for those with a breast cancer diagnosis. There are immense innovations in technology and healthcare, and we have numerous treatment options available to us. We have incredibly educated and well-schooled doctors with extensive training and credentials who are there for us to help us heal and recover. They will get us through to the other side. There are always hope and healing right there for us. Once you get over the initial shock of hearing those three words—"You have cancer"—acknowledge the fear, but do not be crippled by it. Gain mastery over the fear by taking action! Now is the best possible time in history to be healed and get ourselves back into health. And it all starts with you.

While I may never know, at least here on this planet, *the exact moment in time* my breast cancer developed, I do personally believe this: God didn't give me breast cancer, but He did give me that little pinprick that led me to persist and discover my breast cancer early on and then led me to the many positive changes I've made in my life. I wish you all the best as, like Dorothy, you find your power and make your exploration to health. May God bless you!

With that said, I am left thinking about this passage from the Old Testament book of Isaiah, a passage that, yet again, I bumped into "by chance" on my breast cancer journey. And here I want to end this book by sharing that passage with you:

Action Items

Action Items

"For my thoughts are not your thoughts, neither are your ways my ways," declares the Lord. As the heavens are higher than the earth, so are my ways higher than your ways and my thoughts than your thoughts. As the rain and the snow come down from heaven, and do not return to it without watering the earth and making it bud and flourish, so that it yields seed for the sower and bread for the eater, so is my word that goes out from my mouth: It will not return to me empty, but will accomplish what I desire and achieve the purpose for which I sent it."

—*Isaiah 55:8–11*[2]

ACTION ITEMS

ACTION ITEMS

NOTES

Appendices

If you'd like to, remove the following pages that have dotted lines in the margin so you can use them for easy reference and review.

7 Steps to Own and Take Charge of *Your* Diagnosis

MINI MENTION

We have a choice: we can take a positive attitude and face our adversity with fearlessness, head-on. We have a choice to make informed decisions by listening to our doctors and breast friends, doing our research, and diligently seeking out all options available to us. We have a choice to use our adversity to empower us.

Here's how I took charge of my diagnosis—and how you can and will too!

RESOURCE A

LISTEN TO YOUR BODY

If something doesn't feel right, it may very well not be. Be persistent. Listen to your inner voice, your gut instinct. Not sure? Then see your doctor. While there may be some fear in finding out you have an illness, wouldn't you rather catch it early than after it's too late? I thought you'd agree!

GO TO THE DOCTORS

Go to the doctor (and there will be multiple ones and many visits) and *be your own advocate*. While I had excellent doctors, they are busy, so make sure you have questions ready for them. Don't be intimidated if they try to move you quickly out of their office after you waited forever to get in! Think about the detailed questions we ask when shopping for clothes, a home, a car, or take-out food! The doctors you choose will literally have your life in their hands. Do not feel guilty, either, if you feel strongly about getting a second opinion. Healthcare is in part a business; you are the customer, and your business is taking care of *you*!

MAKE SURE YOU TAKE NOTES

While at the doctor, as my mom and best gal pal Anita suggested from my very first doctor's appointment: make sure you take notes. Just like the cover of this book started on sticky notes and ultimately graduated into this, the book you're reading, *be prepared*. We hope it's nothing! But just in case, be ready.

In these last pages I have created a form I used for each of my doctors' appointments. Start there and adjust them as you need with your questions. These notes were invaluable in helping me keep track of the tremendous amount of information that was coming at me and allowing me to compare information from one appointment to another and to assess my options and better understand my diagnosis.

BRING SOMEONE WITH YOU

Make sure, if you can, to bring a friend, family member, coworker, or someone else you trust to your doctors' appointments. This is a person who will help think *with* and *for* you. You may be overwhelmed, as I was, with varying emotions of hope and fear and anxiety. It's important to have someone who can help ask the questions you didn't think to ask, are too exhausted to think about, or are too scared to hear the answers to. I'm just being real; these things can (probably will, at some point) happen!

RESOURCE A

REACH OUT FOR HELP

In the beginning, I knew no one with breast cancer—or so I thought—until I started to open up and talk with other women (and men!). I wanted to know what type of breast cancer they had, what type of surgeries and treatments they chose, and how they are doing now, post-surgery. Initially, I felt embarrassed. It is a very intimate disease. I get it; I was there. But know this: if you open up, *I promise you will find unconditional love and support on the other side.*

GET COPIES OF ALL YOUR MEDICAL RECORDS

Whether MRI reports, X-rays, pathology slides, CDs, hard copy paper reports, or any tests or procedures, get your medical records. It is your legal right! And if you choose to go for a second opinion, you should bring the results with you and likely send them ahead of time. By the time my doctors called to report the results, I often had them—before their call! And, I was ready with my questions. Be proactive in your own care.

RESEARCH, RESEARCH, RESEARCH

From your doctors' appointments to your medical tests, make sure you understand the words and definitions. I can't emphasize this enough. I was overwhelmed with a myriad of terminologies that were completely new to me. While my healthcare providers were excellent, they don't explain everything. Do your research by asking questions of your doctors and going on evidence-based and reputable websites. Doing this gave me control and helped me own my diagnosis and be better informed, and these things allowed me to be prepared for the difficult decisions I faced. (Please see the definitions and resources sections of this book.)

You got this! Welcome to the sisterhood.

RESOURCE A

NOTES

Medical Professionals and Spiritual Support Providers

MINI MENTION

The importance of this list is that you fully understand who your care providers may be, what each does, and how they will impact your journey. And, along with you, how they will integrate and provide a continuum of care from your initial diagnosis to your post-recovery healing—*mind, body, and soul.*

While I have listed them in alphabetical order here, you may likely meet first with your primary care doctor, gynecologist, breast surgeon, and so forth. Certainly, there may be others not included on this list. Throughout this book I provide much more about my experiences with each.

The key, at a minimum, is to be aware and prepared for the support you may need or have available to you. Many, if not all, of the different people in the roles below will be involved in some phase of your care—and they can each be a friend and ally in your journey to beat your cancer. And these are just a few of the roles we thought of—you may interact with even more.

As I went about my research and spoke with other breast friends, I came to find having the proper physical therapy (PT) specialist was integral to my recovery. In fact, I needed more than forty sessions with a specialized PT to be able to raise my arm above my head just as I did before my first surgery, a mastectomy. And, terrified of being under anesthesia (thinking I'd never wake up), having a prayer group pray for me at the exact time of my surgery was comforting.

- Anesthesiologist
- Breast surgeon
- Clinical care coordinator
- Dietician
- Gynecologist
- Medical assistant
- Mind-body therapist
- Nurse practitioner
- Oncologist
- Pathologist
- Patient Navigator
- Physical therapist/lymphedema specialist
- Physician assistant
- Plastic surgeon
- Primary care doctor
- Radiologist
- Radiology technologist
- Registered nurse
- Social worker
- Spiritual support provider (priest, minister, rabbi, imam, etc.)

Be prepared. This will help you make informed decisions.

NOTES

NOTES

RESOURCE B

Words You May Need to Know

MINI MENTION

I came to find that, just as each of us has very different personalities, likes, and dislikes, each person's breast cancer is unique. Breast cancer is the second most common cancer in American women to skin cancer. In the United States in 2021, 1 in 8 woman will be diagnosed with breast cancer; 281,5500 women will be diagnosed with invasive breast cancer; 49,290[1] will be diagnosed with ductal carcinoma non-invasive (in-situ) breast cancer; with an estimated 2,650[2] men diagnosed with invasive breast cancer. While you will speak with your doctors and breast friends, and do your research to learn about your unique diagnosis, here are just a few terms to get you started (in alphabetical order here for organizational purposes only).

- Areola tattoo, 178–179
- Axilla, 279
- Benign, 280
- Bilateral mastectomy, 63
- Biomarkers, 193
- Biopsies, 280
- BRCA gene, 65–66
- Breast implants: saline, silicone, 281
- Breast reconstruction, 281
- Carcinoma, 282
- Chemotherapy, 64

RESOURCE C

Knowledge = Power

RESOURCE C

NOTES

RESOURCE C

NOTES

Tests You May Need to Take

MINI MENTION

When I was first diagnosed, I found myself frantically running from test to test to test. Never having had breast cancer before, I had no idea what these tests were for! Doctors' offices are swamped with patients, and while everyone is doing their best, you have to make sure you do yours. Ask questions ahead of time and *be prepared!*

When I showed up promptly at a couple of appointments, I was told they had to reschedule me because I did not follow the preparation guidelines: things like not eating after midnight or not drinking anything in the morning (four hours prior to the test). I was unprepared because the person who scheduled my appointment failed to tell me, and I didn't know to ask. The pearl here is to ask if you need to prepare in advance for any test you are being sent for.

In a few cases, too, I arrived without the needed prescription for the test. The referring doctor's office either never sent it, or they sent it and it got lost "on the other side" in the receiving doctor's fax machine or email. Thus, I had to sit there waiting, scrambling, often even calling the referring doctor's office myself for the prescription! In a few cases, this delayed the test or it got canceled altogether, and I had to reschedule. Moral of the story: make sure you have a hard copy of the prescription with you just in case!

- Breast ultrasound
- Chest X-ray
- Computed tomography (CT) scan
- Image-guided breast biopsy
- Magnetic resonance imaging (MRI)
- Magnetic resonance imaging (MRI) guided breast biopsy
- Mammogram
- Oncotype DX or Mammaprint aka Genomic tumor testing
- Positron Emission Tomography (PET) scan

Ask questions! Always be prepared.

RESOURCE D

NOTES

NOTES

RESOURCE D

Beyond Your Doctors

MINI MENTION

It became clear to me that, after seeing my OB–GYN, breast surgeon, and then plastic surgeon, that there were still numerous other action items I needed to address. Below, I've identified a few from my experience; you too will likely need these. (Department and service names may vary from health system to health system.)

Make sure, as you contact each department or service, that you write down the names of the people you are speaking with, their phone numbers, and email addresses. Also, you may want to jot down their hours of operation. Get to know everyone! And remember to be patient and kind to all you come in contact with; our health-care systems are overworked. Everyone's trying their best.

RESOURCE E

HEALTH INSURANCE COMPANIES

Both before and after surgery, contact your insurance company to review your plan and ensure you have secured all authorizations for appointments, tests, and surgeries in advance. Write down names of those you speak with and, most importantly, *get it all in writing!* (I address this more in the book.)

BILLING DEPARTMENT

It's also important to meet or speak on the phone with the billing department of each practice or medical facility you visit. I always tried my best to meet people in person. It's nice when you are face to face. If you can't do that, a phone call is fine. Again, always ask questions, and get the person's full contact information—get it all in writing. You don't want additional stress with surprise bills or added expenses.

MEDICAL RECORDS DEPARTMENT

While this takes time and can be cumbersome (also due to HIPPA and compliance regulations), you will have to fill out paperwork to access your records. However, it is your legal right to have *all* paper copies of reports and CDs of medical imaging tests. I found it important to have all my medical records for a myriad of reasons, but most importantly so I could review my results and have questions ready for my doctors when they called to discuss my tests. (I address this more in the book.)

PHARMACY

Get to know your local pharmacist. If you can't easily get in touch with your physician for questions about your medications, your local pharmacist is well versed in answering questions, and sometimes, frankly, even more so than your doctor. (This is an area in which they received extensive training.) Plan ahead so that, if you choose to have surgery, once you are out of the operation, your prescriptions are already picked up and in your home. That's one less task to worry about post-surgery!

DISCHARGE/CASE MANAGEMENT/
HOME CARE (POST-SURGERY)

This is important so that when the hospital discharges you post-surgery, you have all phone numbers for those you may need to contact. While most health professionals call you the day after to check on you, it's important that if you need to reach out to them, you have all proper information. Again, make sure you've planned ahead for your prescriptions, which is one less task to worry about while you are recovering.

Navigating through "the system" is daunting—and being prepared is imperative.

RESOURCE E

NOTES

RESOURCE E

Organizations That Provide Helpful and Exceptional Support

MINI MENTION

I was employed at the time, so I was afforded disability for the six weeks it took me to recover from my mastectomy. And from my initial diagnosis, I had health insurance coverage for most of my doctor's appointments and tests, and I chose to have my surgery locally. However, given the current state of our over-burdened health-care system, you may need a little extra help. Below is an incredible list of organizations that provide support in a myriad of ways that may help as you navigate through your diagnosis.

TRANSPORTATION

Angel Flight East

www.angelflighteast.org • (215) 358–1900

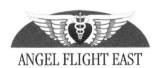

Angle Flight East facilitates flight transportation in the Northeastern region of the United States for distances ranging from 100 to 1,000 miles. They serve the residents of ME, VT, NH, MA, RI, CT, NY, PA, NJ, DE, MD, VA, WV, and OH.

Corporate Angel Network

www.corpangelnetwork.org • (914) 328-1313

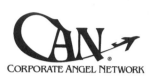

Corporate Angel Network (CAN) helps cancer patients access the best treatment available by arranging free travel on corporate aircraft. Whether a patient is traveling for surgery, clinical trial, or a second opinion, CAN aims to reduce a patient's physical, emotional and financial stress by providing a seat on a corporate flight.

Patient AirLift Services

www.palservices.org • (631) 694–PALS (7257)

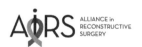

Patient AirLift Services (PALS) arranges free air transportation for individuals requiring medical diagnosis, treatment, or follow-up who cannot afford or are unable to fly commercially. PALS volunteer pilots bear all costs of each medical flight, including fuel, oil, landing fees, ramp fees, and other expenses.

MEDICAL COSTS

Alliance in Reconstructive Surgery

www.airsfoundation.org • (866) 376–6153

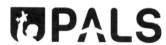

Alliance in Reconstructive Surgery awards grants that will be paid directly to medical providers/facilities to pay for breast reconstruction and related medical expenses. Grants awarded may range from an individual's medical bill co-pay to the full cost of reconstructive surgery, hospitalization, and other related medical expenses.

RESOURCE F

HealthWell Foundation

www.healthwellfoundation.org • (800) 675–8416

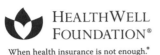 HealthWell provides financial assistance to adults and children facing medical hardship resulting from gaps in their insurance that cause out-of-pocket medical expenses to escalate rapidly; HealthWell assists with the treatment-related cost-sharing obligations of these patients. When health insurance is not enough, HealthWell assists with copays, premiums, deductibles, and out-of-pocket expenses for supplies, supplements, surgeries, and more.

LODGING

American Cancer Society Hope Lodge®

www.cancer.org • (800) 227–2345

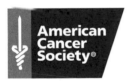 The American Cancer Society Hope Lodges provides free lodging for cancer patients and caregivers traveling far from home for outpatient medical care related to the patient's cancer diagnosis. Currently, there are more than thirty Hope Lodge locations throughout the United States and Puerto Rico. Accommodations and eligibility requirements may vary by location.

GENERAL FINANCIAL ASSISTANCE

CancerCare®

www.cancercare.org • (800) 813-HOPE (4673)

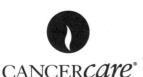 Founded in 1944, CancerCare is the leading national organization providing free, professional support services and information to help people manage

the emotional, practical, and financial challenges of cancer. CancerCare's comprehensive services include counseling and support groups over the phone, online and in-person educational workshops, publications, and financial and co-payment assistance. All CancerCare services are provided by master's-prepared oncology social workers and world-leading cancer experts.

The DONNA Foundation

www.thedonnafoundation.org • (877) 236–6626

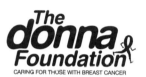

The DONNA Foundation serves uninsured and insured patients all across the country at no charge to help overcome and resolve insurance-related and financial obstacles that impact care. The DONNA Care-Line offers patients diagnosed with breast cancer assistance with access to care issues, insurance denials, workplace and employment protections, medical debt, cost of living debt, and more. The DONNA Foundation also provides education and awareness programs on topics of health, wellness, and living with breast cancer.

The Pink Fund

www.pinkfund.org • (877) 234-PINK (7465)

The Pink Fund provides financial support to help breast cancer patients in active treatment meet their daily living expenses. The Pink Fund grant program helps patients and their families by making payments for critical nonmedical expenses such as housing, utilities, transportation, and health insurance. Payments are made directly to creditors with a cap of up to $3,000 for up to ninety days.

RESOURCE F

NON-FINANCIAL
Cancer + Careers
www.cancerandcareers.org

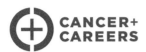

Cancer and Careers, founded in 2001, is a national nonprofit that empowers and educates people with cancer to thrive in their workplace by providing expert advice, interactive tools, and educational events. Its free services include a comprehensive website and library of publications in English and Spanish, legal and insurance information, career coaching, resume review, professional development micro-grants, and national events and workshops for people with cancer and their healthcare providers, coworkers, and employers.

CancerTalks
www.cancertalks.com • (415) 827–5821

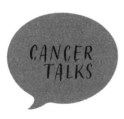

Our mission is to uplift personal stories of transformation from people whose lives have been touched by cancer. Our podcast and blog are open to anyone who has a story to tell. We're building a community of cancer thrivers, and we welcome you to join us. Visit our website for information about biweekly community Zoom calls.

Casting for Recovery
www.castingforrecovery.org • (888) 553–3500

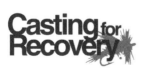

Casting for Recovery (CfR) provides healing outdoor retreats for women with breast cancer at no cost to the participants. CfR's retreats offer opportunities for women to find inspiration, discover renewed energy for life, and experience healing connections with other women and nature. The retreats are open to women with breast cancer of all ages and in all stages of treatment and recovery.

Pink Lotus Elements

www.pinklotus.com/elements

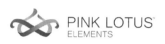 Pink Lotus Elements is a leading online women's health and breast cancer store, shipping to customers in over thirty countries. Shop with peace of mind for a wide selection of functional and high-quality female health products, not pink gimmicks.

Pink Lotus Power Up

www.pinklotus.com/powerup

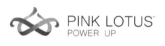 Pink Lotus Power Up is an online social community that empowers women everywhere with resources, articles, news, programs, groups, events, and more. Pink Lotus Power Up's focus is on all things related to breast cancer.

SHARE Cancer Support

www.sharecancersupport.org • (844) 275–7427

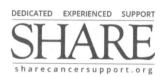 SHARE is a national nonprofit that supports, educates, and empowers women affected by breast, ovarian, uterine, or metastatic breast cancer, with a special focus on medically underserved communities. SHARE's mission is to connect these women with the unique support of survivors and peers, creating a community where no one has to face breast, ovarian, uterine, or metastatic breast cancer alone. All of SHARE's programs are grounded in the needs and insight of real patients and survivors and are developed in multiple languages to support women of all ages, cultures, and ethnicities to make informed, authentic decisions about their health. All of SHARE's services are provided in both English and Spanish, including national helplines, support groups,

expert-led educational programs, community outreach, online communities, corporate education, local advocacy opportunities, caregiver support, and survivor-patient navigation.

Wigs & Wishes

www.wigsandwishes.org/ • (856) 582–6600

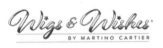

Wigs & Wishes provides individuals battling cancer with free wigs. Salons and stylists throughout the world empower women by providing them with complimentary services that allow them to forget about their fight for a brief moment.

One more reminder: Search for as many local resources as you can find. You may find some cities or townships have their own support centers offering companionship, house cleaning, grocery shopping, support groups, and even scholarships for your children. Sometimes there are simply programs of neighbors helping neighbors.

Reach out for help! You are not alone.
These organizations are here to provide
the assistance you may need.

RESOURCE F

NOTES

Appointments Form

MINI MENTION

While my diagnosis started at my OB-GYN office, for you it may start at your primary care doctor, your GYN, or your breast surgeon. Wherever your journey starts, the important thing is that you are recording details of your visit, asking questions, and taking notes to be sure you're learning about and understanding *your* unique diagnosis.

While it may seem obvious for some, and very generic, this form can be an important source to use to begin to create and build your community of medical professionals in charge of and guiding your care journey. I always do my best to befriend and get as much contact information as possible. If someone is not available, you then have additional contacts you can reach out to. *Remember: you are not alone. We are in this together.*

Note: Make sure to attach this appointment pullout to Resource H: Questions You May Ask at Your Appointments. These will help with relevant questions you will ask each particular doctor.

RESOURCE G

Date and time of visit:

_____

(Know where you are going and make sure to call ahead to confirm your appointment.)

Office address, floor, suite, city, state, zip code:

_____

Office phone number: direct dial and possible cell phone:

_____

Record: Why are you making this visit? Why are you seeing this particular doctor?

_____

The following is important as you complete your office visit forms: they will ask who referred you. Also, if you were referred, you need to check with your insurance company on whether you need a "referral slip" authorization to visit the particular doctor you are going to see. Some insurance companies require referrals; some do not. Do your homework and be prepared ahead of time. Once again, you do not want to be surprised with any additional expenses or bills or be turned away when you arrive (if you didn't get a referral).

Who referred you? Do you need a referral?

_____

Doctor's name, direct phone number, email:

_____

(Several of my doctors would give me their email and, in a couple of cases, their cell phone numbers. So always ask! All they can say is no. Then use the method they have asked you to use in reaching out to them.)

RESOURCE G

Receptionist name, phone number, email:

_____

Care coordinator, phone number, email:

_____

Registered nurse (RN), nurse practitioner (NP), and/or physician assistant (PA), phone number, email

_____

You will not always get the doctor on the phone,
so make sure to befriend your care team while
understanding that their office is very busy.
Be prepared. Be patient.

RESOURCE G

NOTES

RESOURCE G

Questions You May Ask at Your Appointments

MINI MENTION

As I mentioned in the appointments pullout (the previous form), while my diagnosis started at my OB-GYN office, for you it may start at your primary care doctor, your GYN, or your breast surgeon. It's important, regardless of where your journey may start, that you are asking questions and taking notes. You want to be extremely clear on your next steps needed while also learning about and understanding *your* unique diagnosis.

Below are some questions I asked of my doctors along my journey. As I didn't want to make too much of these forms, here's a list of most of the questions I asked of my doctors starting from my first visit at the gynecologist after I felt "something"—that *pinprick*. No doubt you will have many unique questions that may not be on this list, but this is at least a start.

Note: Make sure to attach the appointment pullout (the previous resource) to each of your doctor's visits while noting the relevant questions you will ask at that particular appointment (below). It is extremely important you write down the specific answers you receive. This way, if or when you go for a second opinion, you will be able to ask the second doctor the *exact* questions and then be able to compare notes and make informed decisions.

RESOURCE H

Keep in mind you may not get the answers to all of these questions all in one sitting, and sometimes that is normal. For example, the surgeon may not be able to tell you about chemotherapy options until after you've had a biopsy or surgery. Or, maybe you need another test to see if certain reconstruction is appropriate for your case. There are plenty of reasons why your care provider may say, "I'm not sure yet."

All that said, do try and get as much information as possible from your provider, of course. Just understand that treatment is a process and not every decision can or will be made at once.

- Do I have breast cancer?

- What other tests may I need to assess whether I have breast cancer?

- What stage is my breast cancer, and what does that mean?

- Has it spread to other parts of my body?

- Is my form of cancer of an aggressive nature?

- What are my treatment options?

- What if I chose to do nothing? *Can* I do nothing?

- What are my surgical options? How long is recovery?

- How much disease is there? What is the size of the tumor?

- Do I need radiation? Chemotherapy? Hormone therapy? Other treatments?

- What role do I play in keeping myself well?

- What part does stress, diet, meditation, and prayer play in my life, my current diagnosis, and post-recovery regarding living in the best way I can to heal and be well?

- What is integrative medicine?

- What resources do you suggest I read or go to for additional information on these areas?

- What else can I do going forward to improve my quality of life, facilitate disease prevention, and promote wellness?

- How about my other breast? Is it okay?

- Do I have the BRCA gene? Is my cancer genetic or environmental?

- When do I need to contact my employer/human resources/benefits team?

- What tests or preparations do I need to make pre-surgery?

- What happens during surgery?

- What is a pathology report, and what does it determine?

- If my breast is removed, can I save my nipple?

- What is a lymph node? Do you test my lymph nodes? How many? Why do you test them?

- What about after surgery? What medications may be needed for recovery?

- What other medications may be needed long term to minimize this happening again?

- What treatments, post-surgery, may I need?

- What will I need help with at home regarding various household tasks?

- What is the recovery process like?

- How long will I need for that process?

- Will I need home care support?

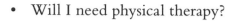

- Will I need physical therapy?

- When will I be able to exercise again?

- What is a compression bra? Do I need to wear one? For how long?

- Will I have scarring? If yes, what can I do to minimize it?

- What kinds of ointments or creams can help minimize and heal scarring?

- What types of routine tests will become part of my annual checkups?

- What is reconstructive surgery?

- When will it be performed if needed?

- If I choose reconstructive surgery, can I determine breast size?

- What types of reconstructive surgeries are there? Risks and benefits?

- What are the options and alternatives to reconstructive surgery?

Be your own advocate.

"The important thing is never to stop questioning."

—*Albert Einstein[1]*

NOTES

NOTES

RESOURCE H

Acknowledgments

As I write this, I'm in a deep place of gratitude. So many people have helped shape this book. Where do I start in thanking them? I have to first start with God. It is unquestionable His hand was upon this project. While we have writers in the family, the passion and drive that has been present in me from that first scribble on that first sticky note until now, six years later, that light that was lit in me is burning ever brighter. To see this through with the same hard-driving, tireless commitment from day one, to seek out and find the answers that may benefit readers, and to see this through to the very last word—that is from above.

Alexandra Duran—lawyer, business coach, and long-time friend—thank you for your wisdom and inspiration. On that very first call, I asked, "Alexandra, what do I do with this? I wrote sixty-three thousand words!" You said I must share my experience to help others. "Your sense of advocacy is powerful. Break it down into chapters. Keep it simple. Be your authentic self," you said. I did just that.

Francesca! You are truly a jack of all trades, an extraordinary designer, therapist, creative thinker, and *breast* friend. For your exceptional cover and interior design concepts, you nail it on the first go-around, every time. What a pleasure it is to work with you; to know you is a great blessing, and your remarkable, angelic patience is simply incomparable. Thank you for accompanying me on this journey.

Sam Salerno, to you and your incredible team at Reel Media. Thank you for your expertise and helping to shine a light on and bring my story to life in such a poignant way to help others. You have an amazing gift. I'm forever grateful for your most generous support, kindness, and warmth in handling such a sensitive, intimate topic as breast cancer with great poise.

Teresa Holliday, my former student, what a serendipitous moment in time for us to reconnect. Nothing, I believe, is by chance. Your extraordinary gifts will benefit many throughout your lifetime and career—for now I was blessed by them. Your fine endnotes and creative sourcing, not to mention your acute marketing and business acumen, are exceptional.

I want to give great thanks to my publisher and his incredible and talented team at Clovercroft Publishing: Larry Carpenter and Shane Crabtree, Lori Martinsek at Adept Content, Solutions, and Suzanne Lawing. For great expertise, guidance, warmth, and grace: thank you. To Bob Irvine, my editor—Bob, someone once told me what makes a great author is a great *editor*. How can I ever repay you? I know! I promise to use less CAPS and *italics* in my next book. Thank you for your superb edits and insights. To Conor Greene, PA-C, my technical editor, I'm grateful for your fact checking, and polishing up of my manuscript to ensure its medical and technical accuracy.

In writing this book, I came across myriad exceptional authors, physicians, humanitarians, healers, individuals,

ACTION ITEMS

ACTION ITEMS

ACKNOWLEDGMENTS

organizations, and resources that are authorities and experts in many areas and fields that are referenced in this book. In Malcolm Gladwell's book *The Tipping Point*, he describes what I have been in writing this book: I am merely the "connector," or the conduit that brought together all these amazing entities and information into one book. This book has been a labor of love, written for all who set out on their journeys after being diagnosed with breast cancer.

I am profoundly grateful to my family and friends, colleagues, and those who serendipitously appeared at just the perfect moment in time and selflessly contributed to help critique ideas and concepts, provide analysis and review of content, offer helpful guidance and feedback, and provide unwavering support and inspiration that kept me pushing forward. I'm especially grateful to Anetta Adamek; Roslyn Aquino, NP; Andrea Aulicino; Vickie Austin, Hallia Baker, CMP, MA, BS; Joseph Binotto; Yuliya Buslovich, MHA; Nella Bastone; Christina Brennan, MD; Patricia Caines, MPA, HHC, CKYT-200; Paul Cantello, MBA; Patty Caruso; Carly Colvell; Margarida Correia; Patricia Delaparra; Patsy Delaparra; Amy Edouard; Christopher Feijoo; Joseph Gargano; Jennifer Grant; Shilo Gold; Nina Hadzibabic, MBA; Sonia Henry, MD; Paula Hoza; Barbara Teitelbaum-Hyatt; Steve Hyatt; Denise Karolewicz, RN; Sheila Keegan, ACSW; Robert Levinson; Yue (Lulu) Liu, MPA, CPC; Denise Lombardi; Christiane Maeder; Adrianna Meza, MPA; Nancy Moszczyski, Victoria Moszczyski, and Gail Murphy; Tara Narula, MD; Michael Pallotta; Maria DeJesus Pimentel; Kyriaki Poumpouridis, MD; Michele Santacroce; Beowulf Sheehan; Francine Smith, MPH; Stuart Tattum; Murray Teitelbaum; Michelle VanVlaanderen; Janice Zaballero; and Justin Zielke, MBA.

ACTION ITEMS

ACTION ITEMS

Finally, to my incredible surgeons and healthcare team: thank you. My deep admiration will always remain for all those amazing breast friends who helped me along my journey to heal body, mind, and soul and got me through to the other side. I'm forever grateful to you.

This book is my way of paying it forward and is dedicated to all those who will be *Just Diagnosed* with breast cancer.

With love,
Arlene

Action Items

Action Items

Endnotes

PREFACE

1 Quote: Toni Morrison: Toni Morrison, "Toni Morrison, Quotes," *Goodreads*, accessed February 4, 2020, www.goodreads.com.

2 Henry Scowcroft, "Angelina Jolie, Inherited Breast Cancer and the BRCA1 Gene," Cancer Research UK, May 14, 2013, accessed April 6, 2020, https://scienceblog.cancerresearchuk.org/2013/05/14/angelina-jolie-inherited-breast-cancer-and-the-brca1-gene/.

3 Rory Cooney, "Jerusalem, My Destiny" (Chicago: GIA Publications, Inc., 1990).

4 Roosa Tikkanen and Melinda K. Abrams, "U.S. Health Care from a Global Perspective, 2019: Higher Spending, Worse Outcomes?," The Commonwealth Fund, January 30, 2020, accessed January 31, 2020, https://www.commonwealthfund.org/publications/issue-briefs/2020/jan/us-health-care-global-perspective-2019.

5 National Center for Health Statistics, "Leading Causes of Death," Centers for Disease Control and Prevention, accessed February 4, 2020, https://www.cdc.gov/nchs/fastats/leading-causes-of-death.htm.

6 Sally C. Curtin, MA, "Cancer and Heart Disease Death Rates, Among Men and Women Aged 45–64 Years—United States, 1999–2018," Centers for Disease Control and Prevention, May 29, 2020, accessed May 30, 2020, https://www.cdc.gov/mmwr/volumes/69/wr/mm6921a4.htm.

7   Infoplease, "Life Expectancy at Birth by Race and Sex, 1930-2010," February 28, 2017, accessed January 31, 2020, https://www.infoplease.com/us/population/ life-expectancy-birth-race-and-sex-1930-2010.

8   CountryEconomy, "United States—Life Expectancy at Birth," accessed January 31, 2020, https://countryeconomy.com/ demography/life-expectancy/usa.

9   World Bank, "United States: Life Expectancy of Women at Birth from 2008 to 2018 (in Years)," Statista, October 2020, accessed November 1, 2020, https://www.statista.com/statistics/263736/ life-expectancy-of-women-in-the-united-states/.

10 Karen Davis, Kristof Stremikis, David Squires, and Cathy Schoen, "Mirror, Mirror on the Wall, 2014 Update: How the Performance of the U.S. Health Care System Compares Internationally," The Commonwealth Fund, June 2014, accessed January 31, 2020, https://www.commonwealthfund.org/sites/default/files/ documents/___media_files_publications_fund_report_2014_ jun_1755_davis_mirror_mirror_2014.pdf.

11 Eric C. Schneider, Dana O. Sarnak, David Squires, Arnav Shah, and Michelle M. Doty, "Mirror, Mirror 2017: International Comparison Reflects Flaws and Opportunities for Better U.S. Health Care," The Commonwealth Fund, July 14, 2017, accessed January 31, 2020, https://interactives.commonwealthfund. org/2017/july/mirror-mirror/.

12 "New International Report on Health Care: U.S. Suicide Rate Highest Among Wealthy Nations," The Commonwealth Fund, January 30, 2020, accessed January 31, 2020, https://www.commonwealthfund.org/press-release/2020/new- international-report-health-care-us-suicide-rate-highest-among-wealthy.

13 "Foundation History," The Commonwealth Fund, accessed January 31, 2020, https://www.commonwealthfund.org/about-us/ foundation-history.

14 Grace Donnelly, "Here's Why Life Expectancy in the U.S. Dropped Again This Year," Fortune, February 9, 2018, accessed February 2, 2020, https://fortune.com/2018/02/09/ us-life-expectancy-dropped-again/.

ENDNOTES

15 Organisation for Economic Co-operation and Development, "About," accessed February 8, 2020, https://www.oecd.org/about/.

16 The British Medical Journal, "About The BMJ," accessed February 1, 2020, https://www.bmj.com/about-bmj.

17 Steven H. Woolf and Laudan Aron, "Failing Health of the United States, The British Medical Journal, February 7, 2018, accessed February 10, 2020, https://www.bmj.com/content/360/bmj.k496.

18 National Institute on Drug Abuse, "Opioid Overdose Crisis," National Institutes of Health, accessed February 20, 2020, https://www.drugabuse.gov/drug-topics/opioids/opioid-overdose-crisis.

19 *Fortune* Magazine, "Ground Zero of the Opioid Epidemic I Fortune," uploaded June 22, 2017, YouTube video, 8:11, youtube.com/watch?v=tYtf5NnyX2Q.

20 Woolf and Aron, "Failing Health of the United States."

21 Woolf and Aron, "Failing Health of the United States."

22 Donnelly, "Here's Why Life Expectancy in the U.S. Dropped Again This Year."

23 Quote: Eleanor Roosevelt, "Eleanor Roosevelt Quotes," Goodreads, accessed February 4, 2020, https://www.goodreads.com/author/quotes/44566.Eleanor_Roosevelt.

CHAPTER ONE

1 Quote: Frankl, Viktor E., "Viktor E. Frankl Quotes," Goodreads., accessed March 8, 2020., https://www.goodreads.com/author/quotes/2782.Viktor_E_Frankl.

2 Cancer Treatment Centers of America, "Breast Cancer Surgery," accessed March 1, 2020, https://www.cancercenter.com/cancer-types/breast-cancer/treatments/surgery.

3 American Cancer Society, "Mastectomy," accessed February 2, 2020, https://www.cancer.org/cancer/breast-cancer/treatment/surgery-for-breast-cancer/mastectomy.html.

4 National Institute of Biomedical Imaging and Bioengineering, "Magnetic Resonance Imaging (MRI)," accessed February 3, 2020, https://www.nibib.nih.gov/science-education/science-topics/magnetic-resonance-imaging-mri.

ENDNOTES

5   Breastcancer.org, (2015), "False-Positive Mammogram Results May Be Linked to Higher Risk Later in Life." accessed February 3, 2020, https://www.breastcancer.org/research-news/false-positives-may-be-linked-to-higher-risk.

6   Cancer.net, (2020), "Computed Tomography (CT) Scan," accessed February 1, 2020, https://www.cancer.net/navigating-cancer-care/diagnosing-cancer/tests-and-procedures/computed-tomography-ct-scan.

7   Mount Sinai, "Lymph node biopsy," accessed February 20, 2020, https://www.mountsinai.org/health-library/tests/lymph-node-biopsy.

8   Johns Hopkins Medicine, "Image-Guided Breast Biopsy," accessed February 5, 2020, https://www.hopkinsmedicine.org/imaging/exams-and-procedures/breast-imaging-procedures/breast-biopsy.html.

9   National Institute of Biomedical Imaging and Bioengineering, (2017), "Mammography," accessed February 9, 2020, https://www.nibib.nih.gov/sites/default/files/Mammography%20Fact%20Sheet%202019.pdf.

10 Breastcancer.org, "Ultrasound," accessed February 9, 2020, https://www.breastcancer.org/symptoms/testing/types/ultrasound.

11 My Breast Cancer Treatment, accessed February 28, 2020, "Understanding DCIS," https://www.mybreastcancertreatment.org/en-US/Understanding-DCIS.

12 American Cancer Society, "Invasive Breast Cancer (IDC/ILC)," accessed February 2, 2020, https://www.cancer.org/cancer/breast-cancer/understanding-a-breast-cancer-diagnosis/types-of-breast-cancer/invasive-breast-cancer.html.

13 Breastcancer.org, "Invasive Ductal Carcinoma (IDC)," accessed February 26, 2020, https://www.breastcancer.org/symptoms/types/idc.

14 Johns Hopkins Medicine, "Invasive Lobular Carcinoma (ILC)," accessed February 26, 2020, https://www.hopkinsmedicine.org/breast_center/breast_cancers_other_conditions/invasive_lobular_carcinoma.html.

15 Cancer Treatment Centers of America, "Common Breast Cancer Types," accessed February 26, 2020, https://www.cancercenter.com/cancer-types/breast-cancer/types.

ENDNOTES

16 American Cancer Society, (2019), "Treatment of Breast Cancer by Stage, accessed January 25, 2020, https://www.cancer.org/cancer/breast-cancer/treatment/treatment-of-breast-cancer-by-stage.html.

17 NIH News in Health, (2017), "How Cancer Cells Spread in the Body," *NIH News in Health*, accessed February 1, 2020, https://newsinhealth.nih.gov/2017/04/how-cancer-cells-spread-body.

18 Quote: Kubler-Ross, Elisabeth, "Elisabeth Kubler-Ross Quotes," Goodreads, accessed March 8, 2020, https://www.goodreads.com/author/quotes/1506.Elisabeth_K_bler_Ross.

CHAPTER TWO

1 Quote: Roosevelt, Eleanor, "Eleanor Roosevelt Quotes," accessed March 8, 2020, https://www.goodreads.com/author/quotes/44566.Eleanor_Roosevelt.

2 The Free Dictionary by Farlex, "Medical Dictionary," accessed March 1, 2020, https://medical-dictionary.thefreedictionary.com/electronic+medical+record.

3 Centers for Medicare and Medicaid Services, "Electronic Health Record," accessed February 3, 2020, https://www.cms.gov/Medicare/E-Health/EHealthRecords.

4 Cleveland Clinic, "Pulmonary Nodules," accessed March 1, 2020, https://my.clevelandclinic.org/health/diseases/14799-pulmonary-nodules.

5 American Cancer Society, "Lymph Nodes and Cancer," accessed March 1, 2020, https://www.cancer.org/cancer/cancer-basics/lymph-nodes-and-cancer.html.

6 Johns Hopkins Medicine, "Breast Reconstruction," accessed February 20, 2020, https://www.hopkinsmedicine.org/health/treatment-tests-and-therapies/breast-reconstruction.

7 Breastcancer.org, "Breast Implant Reconstruction," accessed March 1, 2020, https://www.breastcancer.org/treatment/surgery/reconstruction/types/implants.

8 Breastcancer.org, "Breast Implant Reconstruction," accessed March 1, 2020, https://www.breastcancer.org/treatment/surgery/reconstruction/types/implants.

9   American Cancer Society, "Mastectomy," accessed February 2, 2020, https://www.cancer.org/cancer/breast-cancer/treatment/surgery-for-breast-cancer/mastectomy.html.

10 Breastcancer.org, "Skin-Sparing Mastectomy," accessed February 2, 2020, https://www.breastcancer.org/treatment/surgery/mastectomy/skinsparing.

11 National Institute of Biomedical Imaging and Bioengineering, "X-rays," accessed February 2, 2020, https://www.nibib.nih.gov/science-education/science-topics/x-rays.

12 deBlecourt, Morgan, (2020), "Duke Care Coordinators, Patient Navigators Help You Through Health Challenges," *Duke Health Blog* (June 8), accessed February 2, 2020, https://www.dukehealth.org/blog/duke-care-coordinators-patient-navigators-help-you-through-health-challenges.

13 *The Bourne Ultimatum*, (2007), Director: Paul Greengrass (MP BETA Productions, The Kennedy/Marshall Company, and Ludlum Entertainment).

14 Frankl, Viktor, (1959), *Man's Search for Meaning.* (Boston: Beacon Press, 1959).

15 Yaniger, Batya, (2017), "Logotherapy in a Nutshell," *Psychology Everywhere* (October 18), accessed February 5, 2020, https://www.psychologyeverywhere.com/article/logotherapy-in-a-nutshell.html.

16 Frankl, Viktor, (1959), *Man's Search for Meaning,* (Boston: Beacon Press, 1959).

17 Quote: Frankl, Viktor, "Viktor Frankl Quotes," accessed March 8, 2020, https://www.goodreads.com/author/quotes/2782.Viktor_E_Frankl.

CHAPTER THREE

1   Quote: Edith Wharton, "Edith Wharton, Quotes," *Goodreads,* accessed March 2, 2020, https://www.goodreads.com/author/quotes/16.Edith_Wharton.

2   Johns Hopkins Medicine, "The Johns Hopkins Kimmel Cancer Center Presents: Yoga Nidra," YouTube video, 40:30, April 1, 2015, accessed [date], https://www.youtube.com/watch?v=42fa1BG_MtM.

3 National Center for Complimentary and Integrative Health, "Meditation: In Depth," April 2016, accessed February 3, 2020, https://www.nccih.nih.gov/health/meditation-in-depth.

4 Mayo Clinic, "Integrative Medicine," accessed February 3, 2020, https://www.mayoclinic.org/departments-centers/integrative-medicine-health/sections/overview/ovc-20464567.

5 SHARE, "About Us," accessed March 1, 2020, https://www.sharecancersupport.org/about-us/.

6 Gilda's Club NYC, "Our History & Mission," accessed February 26, 2020, https://gildasclubnyc.org/our-history-mission/.

7 Ken Dembny, "What Is a Capsular Contracture?," *My Breast Augmentation Info,* February 18, 2015, accessed March 2, 2020, https://mybreastaugmentation.info/what-is-a-capsular-contracture/.

8 Pam Stephan, "Capsular Contracture and Breast Implants," *VeryWell Health*, January 6, 2020, accessed March 27, 2020, https://www.verywellhealth.com/capsular-contracture-and-breast-implants-430016.

9 Allen Saunders, "Allen Saunders Quotes," *Goodreads,* accessed March 5, 2020, https://www.goodreads.com/author/quotes/276029.Allen_Saunders.

10 American Cancer Society, "Mastectomy," accessed March 5, 2020, https://www.cancer.org/cancer/breast-cancer/treatment/surgery-for-breast-cancer/mastectomy.html.

11 American Cancer Society, "Radiation for Breast Cancer," accessed March 1, 2020, https://www.cancer.org/cancer/breast-cancer/treatment/radiation-for-breast-cancer.html.

12 Mayo Clinic, "Chemotherapy," accessed February 23, 2020, https://www.mayoclinic.org/tests-procedures/chemotherapy/about/pac-20385033.

13 National Breast Cancer Foundation, Inc., "BRCA: The Breast Cancer Gene," accessed February 26, 2020, https://www.nationalbreastcancer.org/what-is-brca.

14 Operative Neurosurgery, "Jackson-Pratt Drain," Operative Neurosurgery, accessed January 30, 2020, https://operativeneurosurgery.com/doku.php?id=jackson_pratt_drain.

15 The Free Dictionary by Farlex, "Necrosis," accessed March 2, 2020, https://www.thefreedictionary.com/necrosis.

ENDNOTES

16 MedlinePlus, "Gangrene," accessed March 15, 2020, https://medlineplus.gov/gangrene.html.

17 Breastcancer.org, "Tamoxifen (Brand Names: Nolvadex, Soltamox)," accessed March 1, 2020, https://www.breastcancer.org/treatment/hormonal/serms/tamoxifen.

18 Breastcancer.org, "Nipple Reconstruction Surgery and Nipple Tattoos," accessed March 2, 2020, https://www.breastcancer.org/treatment/surgery/reconstruction/types/nipple.

19 Dr. Minas Chrysopoulo, "CT Angiogram Before DIEP Flap Reconstruction—Who Needs It?," *PRMA Plastic Surgery,* accessed May 1, 2020, https://prma-enhance.com/breast-reconstruction-blog/ct-angiogram-before-diep-flap-reconstruction-who-needs-it/.

20 Hospital for Special Surgery, "What Is an Anesthesiologist?," accessed April 8, 2020, https://www.hss.edu/what-is-an-anesthesiologist.asp.

21 The Vinnie Myers Team, "The Vinnie Myers Team," accessed February 16, 2020, www.vinniemyersteam.com.

22 Mayo Clinic, "Breast Reconstruction with Implants," accessed March 4, 2020, https://www.mayoclinic.org/tests-procedures/breast-reconstruction-implants/about/pac-20384934.

23 Breastcancer.org, "Nipple Reconstruction Surgery and Nipple Tattoos," accessed March 2, 2020, https://www.breastcancer.org/treatment/surgery/reconstruction/types/nipple.

24 Max Ehrmann, "Desiderata," in *The Poems of Max Ehrmann* (Boston: Bruce Humphries Publishing Company, 1948).

CHAPTER FOUR

1 Quote: James Thurber, "James Thurber Quotes," *Goodreads,* accessed March 20, 2020, https://www.goodreads.com/author/quotes/16839.James_Thurber.

2 U.S. Cancer Statistics Working Group, "Leading Cancer Cases and Deaths, All Races/Ethnicities, Male and Female, 2017," *U.S. Department of Health and Human Services, Centers for Disease Control and Prevention and National Cancer Institute,* June 2020, accessed June 21, 2020, https://gis.cdc.gov/Cancer/USCS/DataViz.html.

ENDNOTES

3   Peter Criss, "Original KISS drummer celebrates surviving breast cancer," interview by Madison Park, *CNN,* October 15, 2009, https://www.cnn.com/2009/HEALTH/10/15/male.breast.cancer/index.html.

4   Siobhan O'Connor, "Why Doctors Are Rethinking Breast-Cancer Treatment," *Time*, October 1, 2015, accessed March 29, 2020, https://time.com/4057310/breast-cancer-overtreatment/.

5   Michelle Tauber, "Inside Rita Wilson's Breast Cancer Diagnosis and Treatment," *People*, April 14, 2015, accessed March 26, 2020, https://people.com/celebrity/rita-wilson-breast-cancer-inside-her-diagnosis-and-treatment/.

6   Breastcancer.org, "Lobular Carcinoma in Situ (LCIS)," accessed April 18, 2020, https://www.breastcancer.org/symptoms/types/lcis.

7   Elizabeth Sporkin, "My Breast Cancer Journey," *People Magazine,* May 25, 2015.

8   CNN, "Christina Applegate: Why I had a double mastectomy," *CNN,* October 14, 2008, accessed June 8, 2020, https://www.cnn.com/2008/LIVING/10/14/o.christina.applegate.double.mastectomy/.

9   DenseBreast-info, accessed March 18, 2020, https://densebreast-info.org/.

10 Angelina Jolie, "My Medical Choice," *The New York Times,* May 14, 2013, accessed February 23, 2020, https://www.nytimes.com/2013/05/14/opinion/my-medical-choice.html.

11 O'Connor, "Why Doctors Are Rethinking Breast-Cancer Treatment."

12 Quote: Eleanor Roosevelt, "Eleanor Roosevelt Quotes," *Goodreads,* accessed March 20, 2020, https://www.goodreads.com/author/quotes/44566.Eleanor_Roosevelt.

CHAPTER FIVE

1   Health Canada, "Carcinogens in Tobacco Smoke," *Government of Canada*, accessed April 8, 2020, https://www.canada.ca/en/health-canada/services/publications/healthy-living/carcinogens-tobacco-smoke.html.

2   Cleveland Clinic, "Sun Exposure & Skin Cancer," accessed April 4, 2020, https://my.clevelandclinic.org/health/diseases/10985-sun-exposure--skin-cancer.

ENDNOTES

3 Dana Sparks, "Mayo Mindfulness: Stress Effects on Your Body and Behavior," *Mayo Clinic News Network,* April 10, 2019, accessed April 19, 2020, https://newsnetwork.mayoclinic.org/discussion/mayo-mindfulness-stress-effects-on-your-body-and-behavior/.

4 Tim Povtak, "9/11 Cancer Deaths Continue to Rise," *Asbestos.com,* September 10, 2018, accessed April 29, 2020, https://www.asbestos.com/news/2018/09/10/september-11-cancer-deaths-rise/.

5 Henry Scowcroft, "Angelina Jolie, Inherited Breast Cancer and the BRCA1 Gene," *Cancer Research UK,* May 14, 2013, accessed April 6, 2020, https://scienceblog.cancerresearchuk.org/2013/05/14/angelina-jolie-inherited-breast-cancer-and-the-brca1-gene/.

6 Mayo Clinic, "Plantar Fasciitis," accessed June 1, 2020, https://www.mayoclinic.org/diseases-conditions/plantar-fasciitis/diagnosis-treatment/drc-20354851.

7 The University of Arizona Andrew Weil Center for Integrative Medicine, "What is IM/IH?," accessed May 25, 2020, www.integrativemedicine.arizona.edu.

8 Mark Hyman. *The Blood Sugar Solution: The Ultrahealthy Program for Losing Weight, Preventing Disease, and Feeling Great* (New York: Little, Brown and Company, 2012).

9 The Physicians Committee for Responsible Medicine, accessed March 18, 2020, www.pcrm.org.

10 Reference, "What are Refined Foods?," accessed March 12, 2020, https://www.reference.com/world-view/refined-foods -7d8cf6bb22e9640.

11 Georgia Ede, MD, "Beyond Sugar-Free: An Illustrated Guide to Refined Carbohydrates & Insulin Resistance," *Diagnosis: Diet,* accessed April 3, 2020, https://www.diagnosisdiet.com/files/content/promos/refined_carbohydrate_ebook/refined-carbs-ebook-Georgia-Ede-MD.pdf.

12 Hector Sectzer, "The Unhealthy Fats to Stay Away From," *Smartness Health,* accessed March 2, 2020, https://www.smartnesshealth.com/food/the-unhealthy-fats-to-stay-away-from/.

13 Daniel 1:1-16 (American Standard Version (ASV)).

14 Dr. Peter J. D'Adamo, *Eat Right For 4 Your Type: The Individualized Diet Solution to Staying Healthy, Living Longer & Achieving Your Ideal Weight* (New York: G.P. Putnam's Sons, 1996).

15 D'Adamo, *Eat Right For 4 Your Type,* 8.

16 American Cancer Society, "Recombinant Bovine Growth Hormone," accessed May 16, 2020, https://www.cancer.org/cancer/cancer-causes/recombinant-bovine-growth-hormone.html.

17 Neal Barnard, MD, *The Cheese Trap: How Breaking a Surprising Addiction Will Help You Lose Weight, Gain Energy, and Get Healthy* (New York: Grand Central, 2017).

18 Healthline, "Is Dairy Inflammatory?," accessed May 7, 2020, https://www.healthline.com/nutrition/is-dairy-inflammatory.

19 Rodale News, "6 Foods That Cause Inflammation," *Women's Health,* November 21, 2014, accessed March 24, 2020, https://www.womenshealthmag.com/food/a19983367/inflammatory-foods/.

20 T. Colin Campbell, PhD and Thomas M. Campbell II, MD, *The China Study: The Most Comprehensive Study of Nutrition Ever Conducted and the Startling Implications for Diet, Weight Loss and Long-term Health* (Dallas: BenBella Books, 2005).

21 Campbell, *The China Study.*

22 Campbell, *The China Study.*

23 Mark Hyman, MD, "Top 10 Big Ideas: How to Detox From Sugar," *Dr. Hyman Blog,* March 6, 2014, accessed May 15, 2020, https://drhyman.com/blog/2014/03/06/top-10-big-ideas-detox-sugar/.

24 Sophia Lunt, "Starving Cancer Away | Sophia Lunt | TEDxMSU," filmed at TEDxMSU, Lansing, MI, YouTube video, 10:29, https://www.youtube.com/watch?v=f6rSuJ2YheQ .

25 Yella Hewings-Martin, PhD, "Sugar and Cancer: A Surprise Connection or 50-Year Cover-up?," *Medical News Today,* November 24, 2017, accessed May 10, 2020, https://www.medicalnewstoday.com/articles/320156.

26 Maggie Fox, "Here's How Sugar Might Fuel the Growth of Cancer," *NBC News,* December 31, 2015, accessed May 1, 2020, https://www.nbcnews.com/health/cancer/here-s-how-sugar-might-fuel-growth-cancer-n488456.

27 Fox, "Here's How Sugar Might Fuel the Growth of Cancer."

28 World Health Organization, "WHO calls on countries to reduce sugars intake among adults and children," March 4, 2015, accessed May 4, 2020, https://www.who.int/news/item/04-03-2015-who-calls-on-countries-to-reduce-sugars-intake-among-adults-and-children.

ENDNOTES

29 American Heart Association, "How much sugar is too much?," accessed April 25, 2020, https://www.heart.org/en/healthy-living/healthy-eating/eat-smart/sugar/how-much-sugar-is-too-much.

30 Robert Kenner, *Food, Inc.* (New York: Magnolia Pictures, 2008), video.

31 Environmental Working Group, accessed May 8, 2020, https://www.ewg.org.

32 U.S. Food and Drug Administration, "What We Do,"accessed April 15, 2020https://www.fda.gov/about-fda/what-we-do.

33 Campbell, *The China Study.*

34 Campbell, *The China Study.*

35 Centers for Disease Control and Prevention, "A Bold Promise to the Nation," accessed February 4, 2020, https://www.cdc.gov/about/24-7/index.html.

36 Kelly A. Turner, PhD, *Radical Remission: Surviving Cancer Against All Odds* (New York: HarperCollins Publishers, 2014).

37 Lissa Rankin, MD, *Mind Over Medicine: Scientific Proof That You Can Heal Yourself* (Carlsbad, California: Hay House Inc., 2014).

38 Kris Carr, *Crazy Sexy Diet: Eat Your Veggies, Ignite Your Spark, And Live Like You Mean It!* (Charleston, SC: Skirt!, 2011).

39 Bernie S. Siegel, MD, *Love, Medicine & Miracles* (New York: HarperCollins Publishers, 1986).

40 T.S. Eliot, "T.S. Eliot Quotes," *Goodreads,* accessed May 4, 2020, https://www.goodreads.com/author/quotes/18540.T_S_Eliot.

41 Siddhartha Mukherjee, interview by Fareed Zakaria, *CNN,* November 27, 2016, http://transcripts.cnn.com/TRANSCRIPTS/1611/27/fzgps.01.html.

42 Siddhartha Mukherjee, *The Gene: An Intimate History* (New York: Scribner, 2017).

43 Quote: Mark Hyman, MD, "The Missing Link that Keeps You Lean & Healthy," *Dr. Hyman* (blog), November 24, 2015, accessed May 19, 2020, https://drhyman.com/blog/2015/11/24/the-missing-link-that-keeps-you-lean-healthy/.

CHAPTER SIX

1 Quote: Deepak Chopra, "Deepak Chopra Wisdom Quotes," *Pearls of Wisdom,* accessed June 18, 2020, http://www.sapphyr.net/smallgems/quotes-author-deepakchopra.htm.

2 The University of Arizona Andrew Weil Center for Integrative Medicine, "What is IM/IH?", accessed May 25, 2020, www.integrativemedicine.arizona.edu.

3 Johns Hopkins Medicine, "Types of Complementary and Alternative Medicine," accessed May 14, 2020, https://www.hopkinsmedicine.org/health/wellness-and -prevention/types-of-complementary-and-alternative-medicine.

4 Saul Mcleod, MRes, PhD, "Type A and B Personality," *Simply Psychology*, 2017, accessed June 14, 2020, https://www.simplypsychology.org/personality-a.html.

5 Peggy Huddleston, *Prepare for Surgery, Heal Faster: A Guide of Mind-Body Techniques* (Cambridge, MA: Angel River Press, 2012, 2013).

6 Victor Fleming, *The Wizard of Oz* (Beverly Hills, CA: Metro-Goldwyn-Mayer, 1939), video.

7 Fleming, *The Wizard of Oz*.

8 Eleanor Roosevelt, "Eleanor Roosevelt Quotes," *Goodreads*, accessed June 18, 2020, https://www.goodreads.com/author/ quotes/44566.Eleanor_Roosevelt.

9 Rumer Godden, "Rumer Godden Quotes," *Goodreads*, accessed June 28, 2020, https://www.goodreads.com/author/ quotes/2572.Rumer_Godden.

10 Hospital for Special Surgery, "What Is an Anesthesiologist?," accessed June 17, 2020, https://www.hss.edu/what-is-an -anesthesiologist.asp.

11 Huddleston, *Prepare for Surgery, Heal Faster*, 7.

12 Huddleston, *Prepare for Surgery, Heal Faster*, 135.

13 Huddleston, *Prepare for Surgery, Heal Faster*, 135–36.

14 Huddleston, *Prepare for Surgery, Heal Faster*, 110–14.

15 The League of the Miraculous Infant Jesus of Prague, "Novena Prayer to the Infant," accessed June 26, 2020, https://infantprague.org/novena-prayer-to-the-infant/.

16 Johns Hopkins Medicine, "The Johns Hopkins Kimmel Cancer Center Presents: Yoga Nidra," YouTube video, 40:30, April 1, 2015, accessed June 7, 2020, https://www.youtube.com/ watch?v=42fa1BG_MtM.

ENDNOTES

273

17 Kristi Funk, MD, "A Patient's Journey: Angelina Jolie," *Breast Cancer 101* (blog), Pink Lotus Power Up, accessed June 25, 2020, https://pinklotus.com/powerup/breastcancer101/a-patients-journey-angelina-jolie/.

18 Brittanica, "Arnica," accessed June 21, 2020, https://www.britannica.com/plant/arnica.

19 Healthline, "Bromelain," accessed June 7, 2020, https://www.healthline.com/health/bromelain.

20 Michael T. Murray, ND, "5 Ways to Bounce Back Quickly After Anesthesia," *Mind Body Green*, May 28, 2013, accessed June 27, 2020, https://www.mindbodygreen.com/0-9646/5-ways-to-bounce-back -quickly-after-anesthesia.html.

21 Biocorneum Advanced Scar Treatment, accessed June 30, 2020, www.biocorneum.com.

22 Healthline, "7 Health Benefits of Manuka Honey, Based on Science," accessed June 17, 2020, https://www.healthline.com/nutrition/manuka-honey-uses-benefits.

23 Memorial Sloan Kettering Cancer Center, "How to Shower Using Hibiclens®," accessed July 1, 2020, https://www.mskcc.org/cancer-care/patient-education/showering-hibiclens.

24 Catholic News Agency, "Our Lady of Lourdes," accessed June 14, 2020, https://www.catholicnewsagency.com/resource/55431/our-lady-of-lourdes.

25 Quote: Matthew 18:20, https://www.biblegateway.com/passage/?search=matthew+18%3A20&version=NIV.

CHAPTER SEVEN

1 Quote: Angelina Jolie, "My Medical Choice," *The New York Times*, May 14, 2013, accessed July 23, 2020, https://www.nytimes.com/2013/05/14/opinion/my-medical-choice.html.

2 Operative Neurosurgery, "Jackson-Pratt Drain," accessed July 30, 2020, https://operativeneurosurgery.com/doku.php?id=jackson_pratt_drain.

3 Ecclesiastes 3:4, https://www.biblegateway.com/passage/?search=Ecclesiastes%203%3A4&version=NIV.

ENDNOTES

4   Caitlin Kiernan, "A Tattoo That Completes A New Breast," *The New York Times*, June 2, 2014, accessed July 14, 2020, https://well.blogs.nytimes.com/2014/06/02/a-tattoo-that-completes-a-new-breast/.

5   Little Vinnie's Tattoos, accessed July 16, 2020, www.littlevinniesfinksburg.com.

6   Jennifer Whitlock, RN, MSN, FN, "Common Complications and Concerns After Surgery," *VeryWell Health*, January 9, 2020, accessed June 28, 2020, https://www.verywellhealth.com/know-the-most-common-complications-after-surgery-3157301.

7   "Sentinel Node Biopsy for Breast Cancer: What to Expect at Home," MyHealth Alberta, accessed July 7, 2020, https://myhealth.alberta.ca/Health/aftercareinformation/pages/conditions.aspx?hwid=ug3511.

8   John Hopkins Medicine "Lymphedema Therapy," accessed August 4, 2020, https://www.hopkinsmedicine.org/physical_medicine_rehabilitation/services/programs/lymphedema-therapy.html.

9   Rachel Nall, "10 Postsurgery Bras & How to Choose." Healthline, March 17, 2021, accessed March 17, 2021, https://www.healthline.com/health/10-postsurgery-bras-how-to-choose.

10 Breastcancer.org, "Surgical Margins," accessed August 2, 2020, https://www.breastcancer.org/symptoms/diagnosis/margins.

11 Breastcancer.org, "Tamoxifen (Brand Names: Nolvadex, Soltamox)," accessed August 1, 2020, https://www.breastcancer.org/treatment/hormonal/serms/tamoxifen.

12 Memorial Sloan Kettering Cancer Center, "Uterine (Endometrial) Cancer," accessed August 1, 2020, https://www.mskcc.org/cancer-care/types/uterine-endometrial.

13 Penn Medicine Abramson Cancer Center, "Hormone Positive Breast Cancer," accessed August 28, 2020, https://www.pennmedicine.org/cancer/types-of-cancer/breast-cancer/types-of-breast-cancer/hormone-positive-breast-cancer.

14 Webmd.com, "Types of Breast Cancer," accessed August 17, 2020, https://www.webmd.com/breast-cancer/guide/breast-cancer-types.

15 Nutrawiki.org, "Estrogen," accessed August 7, 2020, https://nutrawiki.org/Estrogen/.

ENDNOTES

16 Melinda Ratini, DO, MS, "Progesterone," WebMD, March 3, 2020, accessed August 9, 2020, https://www.webmd.com/vitamins-and-supplements/progesterone-uses-and-risks.

17 Breastcancer.org, "Oncotype DX Genomic Tests," accessed August 11, 2020, https://www.breastcancer.org/symptoms/testing/types/oncotype_dx.

18 Centers for Disease Control, "World Trade Center Health Program," accessed August 14, 2020, https://www.cdc.gov/wtc/.

19 September 11th Victim Compensation Fund, "September 11th Victim Compensation Fund," accessed August 26, 2020, https://www.vcf.gov.

CHAPTER EIGHT

1 Maggie L. Shaw, "Long-Term Risk of Invasive Breast Cancer Increases Following a Diagnosis of DCIS," *American Journal of Managed Care*, May 27, 2020, accessed August 20, 2020, https://www.ajmc.com/view/longterm-risk-of-invasive-breast-cancer-increases-following-a-diagnosis-of-dcis.

2 Carmen J Allegra et al., "NIH State-of-the-Science Conference Statement: Diagnosis and Management of Ductal Carcinoma in Situ (DCIS)," *NIH Consensus and State-of-the-Science Statements* 26, no. 2 (2009): 1–27, https://consensus.nih.gov/2009/dcisstatement.htm.

3 Siobhan O'Connor, "Why Doctors Are Rethinking Breast-Cancer Treatment," *Time*, October 1, 2015, accessed March 29, 2020, https://time.com/magazine/us/4057277/october-12th-2015-vol-186-no-14-u-s/.

4 O'Connor, "Why Doctors Are Rethinking Breast-Cancer Treatment."

5 O'Connor, "Why Doctors Are Rethinking Breast-Cancer Treatment."

6 E. Shelley Hwang, MD, MPH, and Kathy D. Miller, MD, "'Cultural Change': Dialing Back the Discussion and Treatment of DCIS," *Medscape,* January 17, 2018, accessed August 16, 2020, https://www.medscape.com/viewarticle/891198.

7 Gary S. Stein, Janet L. Stein, and Jane B. Lian, "Ductal Carcinoma in Situ: A Brief Review of Treatment Variation and Impacts on Patients and Society," *Critical Reviews™ in Eukaryotic Gene Expression* 24, no. 4 (2014): 281–86.

ENDNOTES

8 O'Connor, "Why Doctors Are Rethinking Breast-Cancer Treatment."

9 Breastcancer.org, "Treatment for DCIS," accessed August 22, 2020, https://www.breastcancer.org/symptoms/types/dcis/treatment.

10 Nancy Hepp, MS, "Clinical Practice Guidelines and Standards of Care," *Beyond Conventional Cancer Therapies*, accessed August 16, 2020, https://bcct.ngo/integrative-cancer-care/clinical-practice-guidelines-and-standards-of-care.

11 Mayo Clinic, "Breast Cancer," accessed August 12, 2020, https://www.mayoclinic.org/diseases-conditions/breast-cancer/symptoms-causes/syc-20352470.

12 WebMD, "Inverted Nipples," September 14, 2020, accessed September 14, 2020, https://www.webmd.com/women/inverted-nipples-causes.

13 Quote: Shakti Gawain, "Shakti Gawain Quotes," *Goodreads,* accessed March 20, 2020, https://www.goodreads.com/author/quotes/41093.Shakti_Gawain.

EPILOGUE

1 Quote: T.S. Eliot: T.S. Eliot, "T.S. Eliot, Quotes," Goodreads, accessed August 20, 2020, www.goodreads.com.

2 Quote: Isaiah 55:8-11, https://www.biblegateway.com/passage/?search=Isaiah%2055&version=NIV

RESOURCE C

1 49,250 will be diagnosed, https://www.cancer.org/cancer/breast-cancer/about/how-common-is-breast-cancer.html

2 2,650 men diagnosed, https://www.cancer.org/cancer/breast-cancer-in-men/about/key-statistics.html#:~:text=The%20American%20Cancer%20Society%20estimates,will%20die%20from%20breast%20cancer

RESOURCE H

1 Quote: Albert Einstein, https://www.goodreads.com/quotes/20604-the-important-thing-is-not-to-stop-questioning-curiosity-has#:~:text=Quotes%20

ENDNOTES

Glossary

#

911 WTC World Trade Center Health Program, health care program for those directly affected by the September 11 terrorist attacks

911 VCF Victims Compensation Fund VCF, fund to compensate victims of the September 11 terrorist attacks or their families, in exchange for agreement not to sue airlines

A

Adjuvant, ingredient used in some vaccines that helps create a stronger immune response in people receiving the vaccine

Anastrozole, drug used to treat early hormone receptor–positive breast cancer

Anesthesiologist, physician who specializes in anesthesiology, which is the application of anesthetics

Anesthesia, drug that causes loss of sensation, with or without loss of consciousness; also, the state of controlled, temporary lack of sensation

Areola, the area of dark-colored skin on the breast that surrounds the nipple

Arnica, herb used for pain, including pain caused by bruises, insect bites, osteoarthritis, and sore throat

Atypia, deviation from the normal or typical state

Axilla, the depressed hollow region located under the shoulder joint, medial to the upper arm; the armpit

Axillary Dissection, procedure in which anywhere from about 10 to 40 (though usually less than 20) lymph nodes are removed from the area under the arm (axilla) and checked for cancer spread shoulder

Axillary Lymph Node Biopsy, biopsy (*see definition below*) of the lymph nodes under the arm

B

Benign, (adj.) that is not cancerous; that is not dangerous or serious

Biopsy, (n.) surgical procedure to remove a small piece of tissue and examine it under a microscope to determine the presence of cancerous cells or other abnormalities; also, the sample tissue itself
(v.) to carry out a biopsy on (someone)

BRCA Gene, abbreviation for **BR**east **CA**ncer (gene), which are two types of genes (BRCA1 and BRCA2) that produce tumor-suppressing proteins; presence of harmful mutations in these genes increase the risk of female breast and ovarian cancers but also of various other kinds of cancer; while most women have a 1-in-8 chance of developing breast cancer in their lifetime, women with harmful mutations in these genes may have as much as a 4-in-5 chance and are more likely to develop cancer at a younger age; men with harmful mutations in

these genes have a higher risk of developing breast, pancreatic, prostate, and testicular cancer

BRCA1, gene that provides instructions for making the BRCA1 protein, which is involved in repairing damaged DNA and thus is tumor suppressing; the BRCA1 gene is located on chromosome 17; harmful mutations in this gene increase the risk of breast, cervical, colon, ovarian, pancreatic, and uterine cancers, as well as "triple-negative breast cancer," a particularly aggressive and difficult-to-treat cancer

BRCA2, gene that provides instructions for making the BRCA2 protein, which is involved in repairing damaged DNA and thus is tumor suppressing; the BRCA2 gene is located on chromosome 13; harmful mutations in this gene increase the risk of bile duct, breast, gallbladder, ovarian, melanoma, and pancreatic cancers

Breast Cancer, disease in which cells in the breast multiply out of control, making malignant tumors that eventually expand locally by invasion and later, systemically by metastasis; there are 5 possible stages (*see* stages below)

Stages, extent of cancer, based on presence and size of tumor and whether it has spread; the most widely used system for staging is the TNM system, in which T refers to the size and extent of the main (or primary) tumor, N refers to the number of cancerous nearby lymph nodes, and M refers to whether the cancer has metastasized (i.e., it has spread from the primary tumor to other parts of the body); each letter is followed by a number (or letter) that provides additional details: for main tumor, TX – it cannot be measured, T0 –it can't be found, and T1 to T4 – refer to size and/or extent; for cancer in regional lymph nodes, NX – it can't be measured, N0 – no cancer (in nearby lymph nodes), N1 to N3 – refer to number and location of cancerous lymph nodes; and for metastasis, MX – metastasis can't be measured, M0 – cancer has not spread to other parts of the body (i.e., there's no metastasis), and M1 – cancer has spread to other parts of the body (i.e., there is metastasis)

Invasive lobular carcinoma (ILC), type of breast cancer that begins in the lobules of the breast, which are the milk-producing glands; invasive means that the cancer has spread beyond the layer of tissue in which it developed and is growing into surrounding tissues, with the potential to spread to surrounding lymph nodes and other parts of the body

Lobular carcinoma in situ (LCIS), unusual condition with no symptoms and that a mammogram doesn't detect, in which there are one or more areas of abnormal cell growth in one or more lobules (the milk-producing glands of the breast), usually more than one; in situ, or "in (its original) place," means that the abnormal growth does not spread to surrounding tissues; even though it is called carcinoma, it is not classified as an actual cancer; however, it increases the risk of future breast cancer

Breast Implant, prosthesis used to alter the size, shape, and contour of a person's breast; used for breast augmentation and breast reconstruction

Breast Implant: Saline, breast implant that is filled with sterile salt water; they are inserted empty, and they are filled once they are in place

Breast Implant: Silicone, breast implant that is pre-filled with silicone gel, which is a thick, sticky fluid that resembles the feel of human fat

Breast Reconstruction, surgical procedure to reconstruct a breast, most commonly in women who had surgery to treat breast cancer; there are two main techniques for breast reconstruction: implant or autologous ("flap")

Breast Reconstruction Using a Tissue Expander and Implant, breast reconstruction technique that involves an expansion of the breast skin and muscle using a temporary tissue expander; after a few months, the expander is removed, and permanent breast implant is put in place

Breast Surgeon, surgeon (usually a general surgeon) who specializes in breast surgery; can biopsy a breast tumor and remove it if it is malignant (cancerous) and can also do breast reconstruction, in which case it is a breast oncology surgeon or a plastic surgeon (surgeons trained in both specialties are known as oncoplastic surgeons)

C

Cancer, large group of diseases characterized by the development of abnormal cells that divide uncontrollably and have the ability to infiltrate and destroy normal tissues; it often has the power to invade and/or spread to other parts of the body

Cancer: In situ (carcinoma in situ), group of abnormal cells that remain in the original place where they developed (they have not spread); they may spread to nearby tissues in the future, becoming cancer; it's also known as "stage 0" disease

Cancer: Invasive, cancer that has spread beyond the layer of tissue in which it originally developed and is invading neighboring tissues

Cancer: Non-Invasive, group of abnormal cells that have not spread outside the tissue where they developed; non-invasive breast cancer is sometimes called carcinoma in situ, pre-cancer, or stage 0

Carcinogens, substance, radionuclide (i.e., radioactive isotope), or radiation capable causing cancer, such as asbestos, tobacco (both smokeless and smoking), cigarette smoke, ultraviolet (UV) radiation (broad spectrum), wood dust, nickel, cadmium, radon, vinyl chloride, benzidine, and benzene

Carcinoma, the most common type of cancer (*see* cancer); it develops in epithelial cells, such as the epithelial tissue of the skin or in the tissue that lines internal organs (e.g., kidneys, lungs)

Centers for Disease Control and Prevention (CDC), national public health institute in the U.S. whose main goal is to protect public health and safety

Chemotherapy, a treatment method that uses a combination of drugs to either destroy cancer cells or slow down the growth of cancer cells

Contralateral, pertaining to, situated on, or affecting the opposite side

CT Angiogram (or angiography), type of imaging test; computed tomography (CT) test that provides detailed imaging of the heart and blood arterial and venous vessels that go to the heart, lungs, brain, kidneys, head, neck, legs, arms, and legs; it uses an injection of a contrast material into the blood vessels; it is used to help diagnosing and evaluating blood vessel disease and related conditions (e.g., aneurysms, blockages)

CT Chest Scan, type of imaging test; computed tomography (CT) test that provides detailed imaging of the organs and structures inside the chest

Compression bra, garment designed to apply pressure to the trunk to keep lymph moving in the right direction

D

Deep Inferior Epigastric Artery Perforator (DIEP) Flap, surgical reconstruction technique in which skin and tissue (no muscle) is taken from the abdomen in order to re-create a breast

DNA, self-replicating molecule composed of two chains that coil around each other forming a double helix; it contains the information for the development, functioning, growth, and reproduction of all known organisms

Downward dog, yoga pose that deeply stretches the back, opens the chest, and builds upper body strength. This posture stimulates the brain and nervous system, improving memory, concentration, hearing and eyesight

Duct, a bodily tube or vessel especially when carrying the secretion of a gland

Ductal Carcinoma In Situ (DCIS), non-invasive cancer where abnormal cells have been found in the lining of the breast milk duct but have not spread outside the duct into the surrounding tissue; it is a very early cancer that is highly treatable

E

Electronic Health Records (EHR), digital version of a patient's medical records, or history

Electronic Medical Records (EMR), a computerized (i.e., digitized) system for maintaining patient health information that generally includes patient's presenting (chief) complaints, history of prior illnesses, prior diagnostic testing, and prior medical treatments

Endocrine therapy, also called hormone therapy, an effective treatment for most tumors that test positive for either estrogen or progesterone receptors

Epidemic, (n.) outbreak of disease that spreads rapidly and affects many individuals in a population within a short period of time; (adj.) that affects or tends to affect a large number of individuals in a population within a short period of time

Estrogen, group of sex hormones whose function is the development and regulation of the female reproductive system and secondary sex characteristics (sexual characteristics not directly involved in reproduction, such as pubic hair growth, rounded hips, and breast development)

Estrogen receptor (ER) positive, type of breast cancer (about 80%) that grows in response to the hormone estrogen

F

Food and Drug Administration FDA, U.S. federal agency responsible for protecting public health by ensuring the safety, efficacy, and security of human and veterinary drugs, biological products, and medical devices; and by ensuring the safety of the nation's food supply, cosmetics, and products that emit radiation

G

Gene, basic unit of heredity made up of a sequence of nucleotides (basic structural units of DNA or RNA); some genes have instructions for making proteins, but many don't

Genetics, branch of biology that studies genes and heredity

H

HER2, growth-promoting protein on the outside of all breast cells

Hibiclens, bacteria-fighting antiseptic used to clean the skin to prevent infection that may be caused by surgery, injection, or skin injury

I

Inflammation, local physical immune response to injury or infection in which tissues become swollen, hot, reddened, and often painful; it can be either acute (i.e., short-lived) or chronic (i.e., long-lasting); chronic inflammation can persist for a long period of time, even years, even after the original trigger is not present; chronic inflammation is linked to many diseases, such as cancer, heart disease, diabetes, asthma, some forms of arthritis, and Alzheimer's disease

Integrative Medicine, approach to restoring and maintaining health by understanding and considering each patient's unique set of circumstances and addressing the full range of not only physical but also emotional, mental, social, spiritual, and environmental influences affecting his or her health

Invasive Cancer, cancer that has spread beyond the layer of tissue in which it originally developed and is invading neighboring tissues

J

Jackson Pratt (JP) Drain, closed-suction, air-tight drainage system placed in wounds during surgery to prevent accumulation of bodily fluids, commonly used as post-operative drain; JP drains promote healing by keeping excess pressure off the incision and decreasing infection risk

L

Lobular carcinoma in situ (LCIS), unusual condition with no symptoms and that a mammogram doesn't detect, in which there are one or more areas of abnormal cell growth in one or more lobules (the milk-producing glands of the breast), usually more than one; in situ, or "in (its original) place," means that the abnormal growth does not spread to surrounding tissues; even though it is called carcinoma, it is not classified as an actual cancer; however, it increases the risk of future breast cancer

Lymph node (or lymph gland), small bean-shaped organ of the lymphatic system and the adaptive immune system; lymph nodes filter substances that travel through the lymphatic fluid and contain white blood cells, which help fighting infection and disease

Lymphatic System, part of the circulatory and immune systems made up of a network of lymphatic vessels, lymphatic organs (including the lymph nodes, the spleen, the thymus, bone marrow, and the tonsils), and lymphoid tissues

Localization, in medicine, describes disease that is limited to a certain part of the body

Logotherapy, psychotherapy developed by neurologist and psychiatrist (and Holocaust survivor) Viktor Frankl based on the premise that the primary motivational and driving force of every individual is the search for meaning in life

Lumpectomy, surgical removal of the breast tumor (the "lump") and some of the normal tissue that surrounds it

Lymphedema, abnormal swelling that can develop in the arm, hand, breast, or torso as a side effect of breast cancer surgery and/or radiation therapy

M

Mammogram, X-ray exam of the breast used to detect early signs of cancer

Mammographic density, a measure of the amount of dense to fatty tissue in the breast; a strong marker of breast cancer risk

Mastectomy, surgical removal of all breast tissue as treatment or prevention of breast cancer

>*Double or Bilateral Mastectomy,* mastectomy (*see* definition above) of both breasts

>*Modified radical mastectomy,* mastectomy (*see* mastectomy above) in which the entire breast is removed, including the skin, areola, nipple, and most axillary lymph nodes, but not the pectoralis major muscle

>*Nipple-sparing mastectomy,* mastectomy (*see* mastectomy above) in which only the breast tissue, not the nipple, is removed

>*Skin-sparing mastectomy,* mastectomy (*see* mastectomy above) that preserves as much of the breast skin as possible; the breast tissue is removed with the nipple and areola

>*Total (simple) mastectomy,* mastectomy (*see* mastectomy above) in which the breast tissue and skin are removed

Meditation, practice that uses a technique, commonly focusing on one's breathing or on the repetition of a mantra, with the goal of reaching a heightened level of attention or awareness and a state of emotional calm and serenity; also, the act of engaging in contemplation or reflection

Metastatic Breast Cancer, the spread of cancer cells (or other disease-producing agent) to other parts of the body from the initial or primary site; also, a secondary cancerous tumor resulting from metastasis classified as Stage 4 breast cancer

Medical Records, document with a patient's medical history, including initial complaints or symptoms, clinical or physical findings, diagnostic test results, and therapies, procedures, and medication used, as well as any subsequent development

Menopause, cessation of menstruation

MRI, magnetic resonance imaging, a medical imaging technique that (through a strong magnetic field, radio waves, and a computer) produces detailed 3D images of the anatomy and physiology of the organs and tissues

>*False Positive,* test result that incorrectly indicates the presence of a particular condition

MRI Breast Biopsy (MRI-Guided Breast Biopsy), breast biopsy (*see* biopsy above) that uses an MRI (*see* MRI above) to guide a needle for tissue removal

Magnetic Resonance Imaging (MRI) Guided Breast Biopsy, see MRI Breast Biopsy above

Monoclonal antibodies, man-made proteins that act like human antibodies in the immune system

N

Necrosis, death of body tissue

Neoadjuvant, of, relating to, or being treatment (such as chemotherapy or hormone therapy) administered before primary cancer treatment (such as surgery) to enhance the outcome of primary treatment

Neoplasm, tumor: abnormal group of cells resulting from excessive cell growth and/or division or from cells that don't die when they should; it can be either benign or malignant

Nipple Reconstruction, surgery to reconstruct a nipple; usually as outpatient surgery and under local anesthetic

Nipple retraction, when the point of the breast turns inward or becomes inverted

Nodule, small lump, or growth of abnormal tissue

Non-Invasive Cancer, group of abnormal cells that have not spread outside the tissue where they developed; non-invasive breast cancer is sometimes called carcinoma in situ, pre-cancer, or stage 0

O

Oncologist, physician who deals with prevention, diagnostic, and treatment of cancer

Oncotype DX Breast Cancer Test, genomic test that predicts a woman's risk of (a) early-stage ER-positive breast cancer recurrence as well as expected benefit from chemotherapy after surgery, and (b) risk of DCIS recurrence and/or risk of a new invasive cancer in the same breast, as well as expected benefit from chemotherapy after surgery

P

Pathologist, physician who interprets and diagnoses the effects and changes caused by disease

Plastic Surgeon, surgeon who performs reconstructive or cosmetic (aesthetic) plastic surgery

Pleomorphic, (adj.) having several shapes; having variable appearance or morphology

Processed Foods, raw agricultural commodity to a procedure such as

GLOSSARY

washing, cleaning, milling, cutting, chopping, heating, pasteurizing, blanching, cooking, canning, freezing, dehydrating, mixing, packaging, or others; unhealthy processed foods have refined grains or added sugar, sodium, or other unhealthy ingredients such as trans fats

Progesterone, female sex hormone involved in the menstrual cycle, pregnancy, and embryogenesis

Progesterone receptor (PR) positive, breast cancer sensitive to progesterone, and the cells have receptors that allow them to use this hormone to grow

R

Radiation Oncologist, physician who specializes in the use of X-rays and radioactive materials in the diagnosis and treatment of disease

Recurrence, if cancer is found after treatment, and after a period of time when the cancer couldn't be detected

Refined (or Simple) Carbohydrates, carbohydrates that have been processed in a way that makes them unhealthy, mainly by adding sugar and/or refining grains (i.e., removing their fibrous and nutritious parts)

Refined Foods, highly processed foods that don't contain all its original nutrients, such as fiber

Relative Value Units (RVUs), measure of value used in the U.S. Medicare reimbursement formula for physician services

S

Scar Tissue, fibrous tissue that forms when normal tissue is destroyed by surgery (or disease or injury)

> *Surgical Scar Tissue,* scar tissue that forms after normal tissue is destroyed by surgery

Serendipity, occurrence and development of happy or beneficial events by chance; obtaining desirable results by accident

Supplements, substances one might use to add nutrients to their diet or to lower their risk of health problems. They come in the form of pills, capsules, powders, gel tabs, extracts, or liquids and might contain vitamins, minerals, fiber, amino acids, herbs or other plants, or enzymes

Surgical Margin, rim of normal tissue that is removed in addition to breast cancer during surgery

T

Tamoxifen, estrogen antagonist used to treat postmenopausal breast cancer

Tissue Expander, implant that acts as a balloon, stretching the skin to make room for the final implant

Triple Negative, means that the three most common types of receptors known to fuel most breast cancer growth—estrogen, progesterone, and the HER2/neu gene— are not present in the cancer tumor

Tummy Tuck, plastic surgery that flattens the abdomen, removing excess fat and skin

U

Ultrasound (Ultrasonography), diagnostic imaging technique (or therapeutic application) of ultrasound (high-frequency sound waves)

Ultrasound Gel warmer, device that warms the gel before it is applied on the skin for application of ultrasound

Uterine (or Endometrial) Cancer, type of cancer that begins in the uterus

V

Vegan Style Diet, diet that only contains plants (such as vegetables, nuts, fruits, and grains) and foods made from plants

Vegetarian, person who doesn't eat meat (poultry, fish, or seafood)

Victims Compensation Fund VCF (September 11th Victim Compensation Fund), fund that provides compensation to victims of the September 11 terrorist attacks (or their families) in exchange for their agreement not to sue the airlines involved

W

Western Style Diet, modern diet characterized by high intakes of red meat, processed meat, pre-packaged foods, candy and sweets, fried foods, high-fat products, corn and high-fructose corn syrup, and sugary drinks, as well as low intakes of fruits, vegetables, whole grains, fish, and nuts and seeds

X

X-ray, high-energy electromagnetic wave that is able to pass through many materials opaque to light, such as body tissues; the photographic or digital image of the internal composition of a body part obtained by using X-rays

Y

Yoga Nidra (or Yogic Sleep), state of consciousness between waking and sleeping induced by guided meditation, which helps relieve stress

GLOSSARY

289

Arlene M. Karole, CHCP

Resources used to date for definitions on this document

Breastcancer.org

CDC Centers for Disease Control and Prevention

Harvard Medical School

Johns Hopkins Medicine

Mayo Clinic

Medical Dictionary (from The Free Dictionary.com)

Merriam-Webster

National Breast Cancer Foundation: www.nationalbreastcancer.org

NIH National Cancer Institute

NIH National Institute of Biomedical Imaging and Bioengineering

RadiologyInfo.org

University of Michigan Medicine

U.S. National Library of Medicine MedlinePlus

GLOSSARY

NOTES

NOTES

Index

An *f* following a page number indicates a figure; a *d* indicates a definition in the text, and a *g* indicates a term in the glossary.

INDEX

INDEX

INDEX

INDEX

About the Author

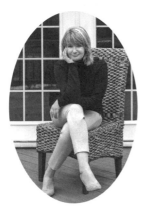

Arlene Karole is a certified healthcare professional (CHCP), lifelong learner, journaler, and educator. She is also the director of the Office of Academic Engagement, Education, and Communications in the Department of Cardiology at Northwell Health. Arlene serves as an adjunct assistant professor at St. John's University in New York City. Based on her personal experience, her book is dedicated to helping others become self-aware and empowered by taking charge of a breast cancer diagnosis. She is active with the SHARE national breast cancer organization, a member of the National Consortium of Breast Centers (NCBC) and on the National Consortium of Breast Centers Conference Survivorship Planning Subcommittee (NCoBC). Arlene has extensive experience working with large health systems and national nonprofits. Her passion to assist others, along with her enthusiasm and commitment to excellence, makes her a sought-after influencer. Arlene has a master's degree in health services administration from Central Michigan University.

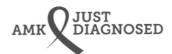

For more information and additional resources visit
www.amkjustdiagnosed.com. A website developed by
Arlene M. Karole to support those diagnosed with breast cancer.

Memorable Moments of My Journey to Healing

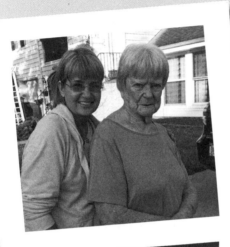

A PLACE TO HEAL
My beautiful Mom provided a place to recover in her home.

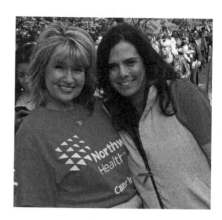

SUPPORT CIRCLE
Breast surgeon, Dr. Jennifer Lehman joined me at breast cancer walk.

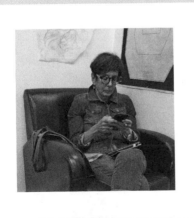

MY BREAST FRIEND
Anita sat patiently in the waiting room during my appointments.